Acupoint *and* Trigger Point Therapy
FOR BABIES AND CHILDREN

A Parent's Healing Touch

Donna Finando, L.Ac., L.M.T.

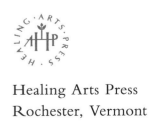

Healing Arts Press
Rochester, Vermont

Healing Arts Press
One Park Street
Rochester, Vermont 05767
www.HealingArtsPress.com

Healing Arts Press is a division of Inner Traditions International

Note to the reader: This book is intended as an informational guide. The remedies,
approaches, and techniques described herein are meant to supplement, and not to be a
substitute for, professional medical care or treatment. They should not be used to treat
a serious ailment without prior consultation with a qualified healthcare professional.

Library of Congress Cataloging-in-Publication Data
Finando, Donna.
   Acupoint and trigger point therapy for babies and children : a parent's healing touch /
Donna Finando.
      p. cm.
   Summary: "Techniques that allow parents to be active agents in providing relief and
healing when illness occurs in their children"—Provided by publisher.
   Includes bibliographical references and index.
   ISBN-13: 978-1-59477-189-7
   ISBN-10: 1-59477-189-8
   1. Acupuncture for children—Popular works. I. Title.
   RJ53.A27F56 2008
   615.8'92083—dc22
                                                                    2007041357

Printed and bound in the United States by P. A. Hutchison

10 9 8 7 6 5 4 3 2 1

Text design by Rachel Goldenberg
This book was typeset in Bembo and Myriad with Warnock as the display typeface

To send correspondence to the author of this book, mail a first-class letter to the author
c/o Inner Traditions • Bear & Company, One Park Street, Rochester, VT 05767, and
we will forward the communication.

To those who preceded me on this wondrous chain of life
offering what they know,
and to those who follow who seek it.
With gratitude and love

Contents

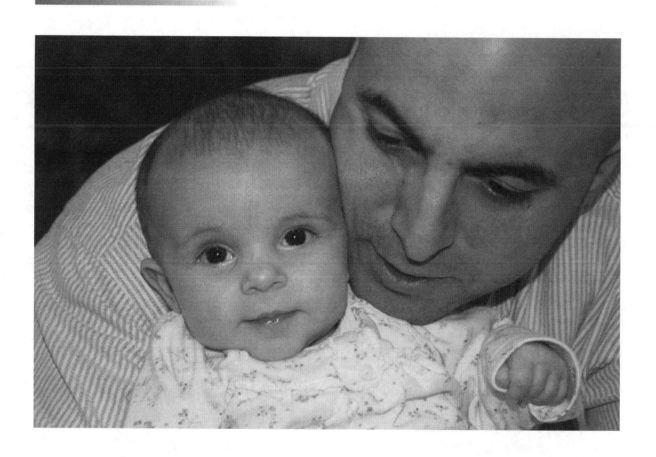

Foreword

Not so long ago I would climb onto my mother Donna's lap when I was feeling bad. At every ache, sniffle, and fever of my early childhood, I would receive soothing touch from her trained hands. There were times when the points she touched were sore, but still I returned to my mother each time I was sick.

As the years passed, the ailments of childhood yielded to the injuries of an athlete. As a wrestler I was plagued with strains, sprains, and all-around pains, but I never missed a match thanks to Mom. There was an additional benefit to these treatments that never occurred to me then; for the time that my mother massaged my various shoulder, back, neck, and knee injuries, we would talk. No modern distractions, just a mother talking to her teenage son while practicing an ancient art and helping me heal. We talked about any number of subjects—I am sure it is a rarity for teenagers to spend the time I did talking with my mother.

In college, wrestling gave way to mountain biking. The miles between college and my childhood home prevented regular visits to my mother, my healer. Often, I would sit in my dorm room in pain and receive telephone direction on how to best massage various injuries.

Graduate school, my first job, a wedding, and my wife's months of morning sickness—all revealing and character-building events in a person's life—shaped me into the adult I am. I have no formal medical training, yet in the months since my daughter's birth I have discovered a unique ability to soothe her, instinctively rubbing her stomach or her feet. I connect with my daughter through touch, just as my mother connected with me.

And now through this book, you can connect with your children as you learn these same healing touch techniques and put them into practice.

Good luck, be gentle, and enjoy your children.

MARK FINANDO

Introduction

As a child I was raised, just as so many of us baby boomers were, by parents who were smitten by the wonders of modern medicine. Initially developed to treat wounded soldiers, penicillin came into common usage during World War II, 1939–1945. Prior to the breakthrough of penicillin for treating bacterial infections, what would be considered common innocuous infections now could easily have been the cause of death.

Childhood diseases were a common and expected trial for every child; mumps, measles, chickenpox, and rubella were suffered equally by most. Some suffered more. Polio terrified parents of small children, since not only was it commonplace, but the damage it could cause ranged from muscle pain and weakness to debilitating paralysis. All of this began to change in the mid 1950s with the development of childhood vaccines, now a routine part of a child's health care.

When I was young, medical doctors still made house calls to take care of those who were sick, something that is now either completely unknown or thought to be a quaint anachronism to most young parents reading this book. If a child were sick, the doctor would come to your home, carrying his black doctor's bag (does anybody even know what that is now?). He'd listen to your breathing with a stethoscope and give you a shot: the magic penicillin. The healing process would begin; parents would heave a sigh of relief.

For parents of small children at that time, modern medicine really was a wonder.

As a child I was drawn to work with my hands. My initial training in the healing arts was in the art of Amma, a sophisticated application of acupressure. My teacher, Tina Sohn, learned Amma from her Korean grandmother. She talked about Amma's ability to ease discomfort and heal disease.

Having been raised under the aura of modern medicine, I was a bit skeptical, until I began using Amma myself, on my three-month-old son. I was amazed at its impact. With a little bit of hands-on work, nasal congestion would clear, a cough would break up and the baby would breathe better, his fever would go down, his ear infection would disappear. Sometimes the cold would blossom after a treatment, but it would come and go in a matter of just a couple of days. The more I used Amma the more I recognized the magic—the miracle of the body healing itself. This was the beginning of what has evolved into a thirty-two-year practice in health care.

As an acupuncturist and practitioner of massage I have had the great benefit of being trained in many elements of two great models of health: one based on Oriental principles, the other being in the Western model of "conventional" health care. My years of practice showed me that not only does each model have its place in health care, but when used as partners they are a remarkably powerful tool, one that spurs the body's ability to heal itself. The information and treatments provided here are the results of the marriage of these two models.

The human body is astonishing. The body *is* capable of healing itself, and with a bit of help—often not very much—it will do so remarkably efficiently. The treatments in this book provide that help. They aren't a substitute for medical care; rather, they are an adjunct. There are times when the diagnoses that are provided by our physicians are essential, and the medications necessary. But there are many times when we know that a cold is just a cold and that constipation is a temporary discomfort that will pass.

Whether or not diagnoses and medications are needed, a hands-on treatment will advance the healing process and soothe a child in distress. The bonus is twofold. First, as a parent you can be proactive in your child's healing regardless of his age. What could be more wonderful than that? Rather than simply waiting for your child to get better, you can help. Second, while you are touching your child, focusing on him, working on him, you are bonding with him. You are deepening your loving moments of connection that feed your relationship and your hearts.

The treatments I include in this book are based on the Oriental model of health care. That system views the body as an integrated whole. It holds that there are meridians or pathways that lie on the arms, legs, torso, and head. Life force energy, *qi* (sometimes spelled *chi*), runs through these pathways. Each pathway is connected with an internal organ or system that functions in our body. (The details of this system are discussed in the An Introduction to Meridian Theory chapter.)

The principle behind this model, simply put, is that when there are obstructions to the free flow of qi through these pathways, that obstruction will reflect in the body as illness and disease. By removing the obstructions the body will begin to heal itself. Massage, acupressure, acupuncture, and the application of heat at specific points are some of the means by which these obstructions can be corrected. This system has been used successfully for thousands of years to treat disease and maintain general health.

The other aspect of these treatments is the massage of the musculature. We all know, even if it is somewhat intuitive, that a hurt always feels better when you rub it. It's instinctive to touch a painful area. Why? The musculature that is related to a particular organ or system gets tight when it is not functioning properly. Which came first: the muscular restriction or the organ dysfunction? It's a good question—from a physiological standpoint, causality may work in either direction. Sometimes restriction in the musculature leads to the organ dysfunction; sometimes it's the other way around. But the bottom line is that when you have a cough, the muscles of your upper body get tight. When you massage your chest and upper back and release the muscles, you start to feel better. You breathe more easily. Ask anyone with asthma. When you're constipated and you rub your belly, it helps. The bowels are stimulated, gas is passed, and discomfort begins to be relieved.

This approach, then, is a combination of acupressure and muscular massage. Anyone can do it. Clear diagrams will guide your hands to where you must touch. I have also included the descriptions of the meridian pathways, points, and muscles that are used in the treatments for those who are interested in the detailed specifics behind these healing practices. The only thing you *need,* however, to promote healing is the desire to help your little one, the willingness to spend time looking into his eyes and smiling at him "face to face, heart to heart," while you gently touch his body.

I have been a health care practitioner for more than thirty years. My years of practice spanned the years in which my son grew from a baby into a man with a family of his own. When I treated him the health care practitioner in me felt great pleasure in helping a child; but the mommy in me treasured those moments together. They are moments that I remember clearly even now and with a smile on my face—lovingly laughing, playing, touching, soothing, *helping* my little one.

It continues to this day.

PART 1

THE BASICS

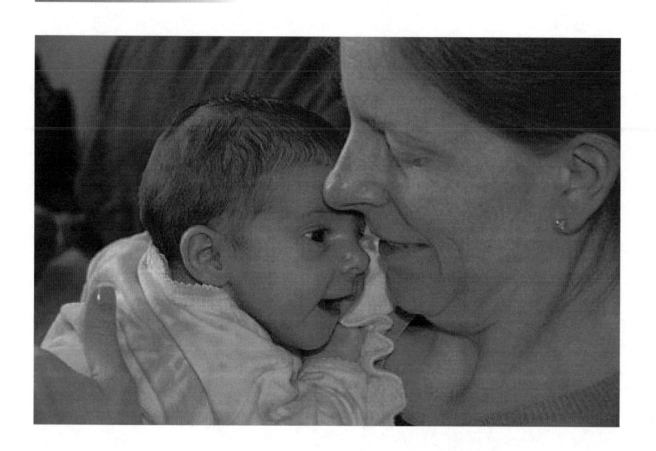

Moments of Bonding

The Importance of Touch
and the Use of Your Hands

What could be more natural than touching your baby? She is a part of you. She came through and from your body. She is a product of your love for your partner. Holding, touching, cuddling is the most natural of a parent's instincts. Through touch we calm and are calmed; we soothe and are soothed; we bond; we connect; we affirm our oneness.

Throughout the ages mothers and fathers have reached out to "rub the hurt" of their little one; to make it all better; make it go away. We seek to hold a crying child and help him. That ache that a mother feels at the sound of her baby crying is the need to soothe her little one.

That's what this book is all about. We are reaching out to touch our children, to help them heal from what ails them.

Babies and small children are amazing. Their bodies do not yet house the areas of tightness, the muscular tensions, that the body takes on as we get older. When we treat an ailment through touch their bodies respond quickly and their bodies retain the treatment. Any areas of muscular tightness that do develop soften right away. A little bit of work goes a long way with a little one. It serves as a reminder that, used with *intention* and *direction,* touch is a very powerful tool: a beautiful, tender, powerful tool.

That tool, quite literally, lies in your hands. Your hands are the agents of touch, and touch is one of the most potent ways that one human being experiences connection to another.

In this book, I offer treatments in which touch is used as the means to help ease the symptoms and speed recovery from those conditions and problems that children most commonly experience. Colds, coughs, asthma, constipation, diarrhea, and common infections of childhood are treated with acupressure using the meridian approach of Oriental medicine. Channels, or meridians,* create a living web within our bodies, connecting the body's surface with the internal organs. A dysfunction in an organ will be reflected in the related meridians as well as in the muscles and connective tissue that lie within and form the pathways of the meridians. For example, let's say you develop bronchitis. You will be coughing; your lungs and your breathing will be affected. The meridians that pass through the lungs will also be affected, as will the muscular areas through which the meridians pass. In this case, those areas are the arms, chest, and back. From the Oriental standpoint, you do not separate the organ, its related meridian, the energy that moves through that meridian, and the areas of the body through which the meridians pass. Rather than seeing the organ, in this case the lungs, as separate and distinct from the energy and pathways that serve and feed it, the whole organ/energy/pathway system is considered and treated as one entity. This relationship explains why you might treat the arm to help the lungs.

The final chapter on children's conditions offers treatments for the various muscular aches and pains that children occasionally suffer. These treatments use massage and pressure to release tight bands of muscle and the trigger points that develop when a muscle is strained. Trigger points are like little knots that develop in the muscles from overuse or injury. Our young athletes most often need this kind of muscular work: our dancers' legs and backs, our pitchers' shoulders and arms, our basketball players' thighs, knees, and legs, and our runners' legs and ankles.

In addition to muscular overuse, trigger points may develop in the presence of disease. For example, the child (or adult for that matter) who suffers a recurrent respiratory disease such as asthma, will very often develop trigger points in the muscles of the chest, neck, and upper back. Again, the whole system is affected. Whether it is couched in the language of meridian theory or in the language describing muscular restrictions, we are, indeed, talking about the same thing. Organs and muscles affect one another.

---

*The terms *channel* and *meridian* are used interchangeably within this manual.

Hands-on work is of great value even if your child is free of illness or muscle tightness. Working on him helps keep him healthy. It helps to prevent him from getting sick and his muscles from becoming injured. If he tends toward getting colds, work on him to open up the musculature on his neck, chest, arms, and upper back. If he tends toward coughs or asthma, work on his arms, chest, and back. If digestion is his weak point, his belly, his back, and his legs will need the most attention. If he's a tennis player, work on his arms and shoulders. If he's a runner, work on his hips, back, and legs. If he's a bit stressed, work on his back and chest. I'm sure you get the idea.

How will you know where to touch? Diagrams and explanations offered for each treatment will guide you, and your hands will tell you. When you touch your child you will feel some areas that are tighter than others. Some areas may just feel thick; some areas may feel ropey; some areas may feel hollow. It's the thick and ropey areas that need the most work. Picture water flowing through a garden hose. When the garden hose gets pinched, the area above the pinch feels thick with water; it's hard to squeeze. The area below the pinch feels hollow and it's easily squeezed. The idea is basically the same as concerns the body: blood, body fluids, and qi aren't moving easily through the area that is restricted. Massage and acupressure will help to soften the area. Restrictions will be removed. The result will be an opening of the flow of qi, blood, and fluids, their free movement being the necessary condition of health.

Treating your baby or your child really can be a pleasurable time for both of you. But first you have to get yourself ready. When you work on your little one you'll use the pads of your fingers or an edge of your finger, rather than your fingertips. Your hands should be clean and soft and your nails short and smooth. Long nails can get in the way, so it's best to trim your nails and make sure that there are no sharp edges; it's easy to harm that delicate skin, even with a hangnail. Then—this is the really important part—make sure that *you* are relaxed. Your stresses, your strains, your emotions come through your hands. Set aside a period of time when you can let go of the stresses of the day and just focus on your child, giving her your full attention. You won't need more than fifteen or twenty minutes for a treatment session.

These treatments are both therapeutic and preventative. They can be used at every phase of life, whether your child is a baby, a youngster, an adolescent, a young adult, a married man, or a father himself. It's easiest to work on a very tiny baby or a child who is old enough to lie still and relax. It's those years in between that can be the greatest challenge. For the child six months to two years old, plan on making treatment time a game. You may have to hold the baby and walk around while you work on his back, or pretend to tickle him while you're actually working on his belly. Working on their hands and arms, feet and legs may be interrupted by a little game or some other distraction. Relax and give time to your child. I've treated my share of little ones while I was walking around the treatment room, holding a baby on my side while turning the light on and off or pointing out the colors or letters on the charts on the walls, and even while reading to them.

Remember, there's no rush. There's no formal way this has to proceed. All you want to do is make sure that you've treated all the necessary areas. Sometimes when Mark was sick with a cold as a small child, I'd treat him throughout the day. If I was holding him I'd work on the points on his arms or his legs. If I was getting him ready for a nap, I'd work on his chest. If he was giving me a big hug, I'd work on his back. By the time his bedtime came, I'd covered all the areas that needed to be taken care of to help him get over his cold. I was touching him throughout the day, taking care of him throughout the day. Most of the time he didn't really know what I was doing. To him it felt good and it helped. I knew it would. Ultimately, so did he.

In the treatments that follow, both verbal descriptions and drawings will identify where to touch. Treatment areas are illustrated using two levels of shading. The lightly shaded areas need some attention, but not a lot; work on those areas once or twice in the course of a treatment. The darker areas need the greater amount of attention. You'll need to work on those areas three or four times during a treatment. These areas cover the region in which an acupoint can be found. (A point is the size of the head of a pin and the area is the size of the pad of your finger.) When you work on a baby or small child, there really is no need to look for the specific point. Their bodies are so receptive to treatment that working on a general area will produce the desired result.

When you treat an area, such as the front of the arm* or the chest, your fingers will make small circles on the skin, like spirals, beginning

---

*The phrase "front of the arm" refers to the standing position when the arms are at the sides and the palms are facing front. In this position your pinky fingers will be closest to your thighs. The phrase "back of the arm" refers to the area of the arm that is facing back in this standing position.

at one end of the area and working toward the other. You should use about the same amount of pressure as you would when you rub an infant's back to help him burp. Little bodies are very sensitive—you won't have to touch very hard. Babies and children are as soft and supple as rising dough. You want your touch to be just as gentle. The pressure that you'll have to use can be very light. Your touch will be just hard enough to feel and move the muscle in that pudgy little body. It's really a very gentle touch. You'll use about the same level of pressure as you would use if you were testing a cake baking in the oven to see if it was ready, or touching something you've recently painted to see if it is dry. Your fingertips barely get compressed. With that level of pressure the baby won't feel any discomfort.

When your children are older than six or seven and their muscles are well developed, you can start to look for specific acupoints. But you don't want to go "poking around." When you find a specific point, your finger will fall into a small hollow or depression. All you need to do is to press lightly into that hollow with the edge of your finger, just enough to gently compress it. It might feel somewhat tender, so don't press too hard. (Of course, most kids will let you know clearly if you're pressing too hard!) You'll feel a slight giving way of the skin and muscle under your finger. Compress the point gently. Feel the child's skin and her pliable muscles under your fingers and hands.

In older, more strongly developed children, and in teens and adults, you might encounter an area of a muscle that seems to be tighter than the surrounding tissues. In order to help it to release, compress it just hard enough to feel the muscular resistance push back under your fingers. Don't try to force an area of tightness to let go: it won't release. It will just hurt, and sometimes those areas can be very tender. When you are working to release a trigger point, if you press it for a few seconds it will start to soften and give way. Be patient. Relax. Keep holding the point. You may notice that your fingers may start to move along with the tissues under them as the tissues begin to soften. I call this the "dance of the tissues." When this happens you can begin to feel how alive and responsive the body is; and you can really feel how touch connects us.

When you work on your child, put your awareness in your hand, feel what it is touching. Feel the connection between you, physical and otherwise. Look at your child. Smile. Talk. Play. Touch. A treatment can be an easy, fun, relaxing time for you both. If your child is fussy and cranky and not relaxing or if he doesn't want to be touched just then, let it go. If *you* are stressed, or distracted by your other children, phones, or whatever, let it go. There will always be some time later, a time that will be better for both of you.

Figure out what works best for you and your child. That will change through the years. The way you treat a baby is very different from the way you treat a five year old or a fourteen year old or a young man in college. You know your child. You'll figure out what and when is the best time to treat. Follow your heart. Intuition and instinct have a place at this table as well.

If your curiosity includes the desire to understand a bit more about the Oriental model of health care, read through the chapter that follows. It contains a description of the basic principles and dynamics upon which the system is based. Fundamental terminology is defined and basic interrelationships explained. I've tried to make the information as accessible and readable as possible for everyone—whether or not you have any background in the healing arts. Getting a sense of the relationships between meridians and organs, muscle and fascia allows you to glimpse the interconnectedness of the structures within our bodies. It explains why touching a lower leg will help the digestive tract, or how touching the arm will help to ease breathing.

While this information might be interesting to some of us, it isn't necessarily interesting to all of us. So if you have no interest in the dynamics of the system, feel free to skip it. A loving hand touching your child with the intention of helping him heal is far more important than all the information in all the books. You don't need details to see that a physical body is a beautiful, interconnected whole that is highly responsive to a caring, healing touch.

An Introduction to Meridian Theory

How many times have I picked up a book and my first reaction to seeing some technical or unfamiliar language was, "Forget it. I can't understand this." I'm guessing that my reaction is pretty similar to many others. So I would not be at all surprised if there are some of you looking at this section, seeing the phrase "meridian theory" and thinking that you should close this chapter now. Oriental healing principles may be new to you. But you might find the basic principles easier to understand than you may think. Every area of study has words that are unfamiliar and may seem somewhat daunting to those who, at first, have no experience with the field. This is true for every field of endeavor from knitting to computer science. If you care to delve in, read the material slowly. The ideas underlying Oriental medicine are fascinating.

You may already know that the Oriental healing arts are amazingly effective. They've been in continual use for thousands of years. Perhaps you'd like to understand a bit more about how and why Oriental medicine works. Whether you've had experience with all this or not, let me invite you all to read on. I've tried to make these basic principles readable to those of you who have the interest.

The Oriental approach to health care is a bit of a curiosity to the Western mind. More and more people are using it and are finding that disorders are being eased if not healed, and yet they are uncertain as to how it works.

Modern medicine as we know it in the West is rooted in the principle of reductionism: if we break everything down into the smallest possible parts we will be able to understand it. The focus is on disease. When disease occurs, symptoms are identified and each one gets treated, sometimes by separate doctors. Problems are often not looked at within the context of the whole system.

The basic tenets of the Oriental model are diametrically opposed to this "pieces and parts" approach. Oriental medicine views the human body as a unified whole, a system in which balance is the primary condition of health. When the system as a whole is in a state of balance, health exists; when there is an imbalance within the mechanism, disease or dysfunction exists. The Oriental medicine practitioner seeks to identify imbalances and correct them to restore health.

The Meridians

Oriental medicine has identified the meridian system, a highly intricate web of interconnecting channels, or pathways, within the body. Meridians pass on and through the surface of the body and penetrate its depths, connecting with one another as they do so. These pathways move through muscle and tissue, connecting the surface of the body to each organ within.*

It is along these pathways that qi flows. What is qi? It is energy, the force of life. While we cannot see qi, we can see its manifestation in the ongoing, unceasing movement that is required for a state of health to exist: the unimpeded flow of blood and body fluids, unimpaired nerve transmission, free movement of muscles and joints, unrestricted digestion and elimination, and the free expansion of our lungs. Rather than being a substance, qi can be thought of as the unconstrained movement of all substance. Look at a healthy child—he is unstoppable, he never sits still. His eyes gleam. He radiates energy. His body is

---

*Interestingly, the description of the interconnection of the meridian pathways is similar to one of the most amazing structures of the body, the connective tissue. Taken as a whole, the connective tissue (or fascia) forms a single continuous sheath within and through body. Connective tissue is the matrix, the ground substance, that surrounds all other structures. Like the meridian system, the fascia "begins" at the surface of the body (as with any continuous system, there really is no beginning), just underneath the skin that covers the body as a whole. The fascia wraps each body part in its entirety, as well as each muscle group, muscle, and individual muscle fiber. It travels seamlessly into the depths of the torso to enwrap and protect each individual organ. It provides a continuous surface upon which nerves and blood vessels lie. In the words of John Upledger, it is "a maze which allows travel from any one place in the body to any other place without ever leaving the fascia." (John Upledger and Jon Vredevoogd, *Craniosacral Therapy* [Seattle: Eastland, 1983], 239)

growing. He is in an all-systems-go mode. He might get sick, but he recovers quickly.

Compare that image to one of an elderly man. He might be active for his age, but he struggles to get through the day without discomfort, pain, or digestive difficulty. He needs to rest often. As the body ages and declines, the systems slow down and energy, qi, wanes.

Perhaps this comparison will clarify: the force of life lies in, and is perhaps reflected by, the body's ability to move all that needs to be moved freely and easily. When movement is impeded by aging or disease, health is impeded: life is impeded.

For those of us who seek to have a material notion of how the meridian system works, it seems apparent that what we are doing when we contact a point on the surface of the body is stimulating this *movement* of blood, lymph, and electrical impulse through the nervous system, through pathways that are carved by the fascia and defined by the meridians. (For a broader discussion see Finando and Finando, *Trigger Point Therapy for Myofascial Pain* [Rochester, Vt: Healing Arts Press, 2005].)

Fifty-nine channels have been defined—the channels interconnect with one another as they wend their way through the body. The meridians comprise a complex system, but one that can be easily imagined. Picture an extensive system of garden hoses. When there is too much water in one part of the system because of a restriction somewhere along its length, there isn't enough in the other part. You have to release the restriction in order for water to flow through the whole system properly. This simple metaphor for the energy system explains why we treat various parts of the body to affect a change somewhere in the system.

The practice of Oriental healing methods involves stimulating points along these meridian pathways. Points on each pathway perform certain functions, and might be stimulated based on that function. Points might also be used based on their location; a point located on the stomach, for example, might be used to treat discomfort relating to digestion.

Points are used alone or in combination to achieve particular results. The reasons for their choice are extremely varied and are often based on the cumulative experience of untold numbers of practitioners over the centuries that acupuncture has been in use. Volumes have been written on it. Seasoned practitioners continue to develop their own compendium of preferred points and point combinations, and so the living healing tradition evolves.

An ingenious measuring system allows for the location of specific acupoints. Each body part is divided into a specific number of *tsun,* or "body inches." One tsun is measured as the length of the second phalange (the center link of the three little bones that make up the middle finger) of the middle finger or the width of the thumb of the person who is being treated. When the four long fingers of the hand are placed beside one another, their combined width equals 3 tsun.

Spleen 6, for example, is positioned 3 tsun above the inside anklebone. When you treat, measure your patient's four fingers together to find the measure of 3 tsun. Place that measurement at the inside anklebone and you'll find Spleen 6.

A baby's four fingers together may be equal to one or two of your own. Keep this in mind when you are treating a baby or small child and trying to locate points. That being said, for infants and small children, their bodies are so receptive to treatment that if your fingers generally cover the area where the point is located, your touch will likely have its desired effect.

The Meridians or Organ Channels and Their Sphere of Influence

Each meridian, or channel, is related to a specific organ over which it has influence and through which it passes. It has influence over the organ's function, and also holds sway over certain characteristics that, to the Western mind, may not seem to be related to that organ at all. For example, the Heart meridian is not only related to the functioning of the heart, but to such apparently unrelated aspects and functions of the human body as consciousness, sleep, and memory. Each organ of the body is also related to a sense organ; the heart and the Heart channel, for example, are related to the tongue. Unusual? Perhaps. However, when a fetus is developing within the mother's womb, the heart and tongue develop from the same formative tissues. It is unknown how the ancient healers concluded this thousands of years ago.

Organs are grouped into two categories. The yin organs, considered to be the solid organs, function continuously: those organs are the lung, spleen, heart, kidney, liver, and pericardium. The yang organs, the hollow organs, function intermittently; those organs are the colon, stomach, small intestine, bladder, gall bladder, and triple warmer.

Yin organs produce, transform, regulate, and store fundamental substances, such as qi, blood, and fluids. Their functions are directly related to maintaining balanced functioning, or homeostasis, within the body. One cannot live without the ongoing activity of each of these organs.

Yang organs receive, break down, and absorb any part of food that is to be utilized by the body, and they transport and excrete any unused portion. Yang organs work intermittently, not continuously—for example, the stomach is not working when there is no food in it.

Each yin organ is paired with a yang organ. The pathway associated with one intersects with the pathway and the organ of the other. Their functions are linked. For example, the Arm Great Yin Lung Channel and the Arm Bright Yang Colon Channel are paired. Functionally, both are involved with water metabolism. A dysfunction in one will ultimately affect the other.

Three yin and three yang channels lie on each side of the upper body and torso and three yin and three yang channels lie on each side of the lower body and torso, each side mirroring the other. As there are pairings between yin and yang organ channels, there are pairings between upper and lower channels. So, for example, Arm Great Yin Lung channel is related to and connected to Leg Great Yin Spleen channel.

The continuous cycle of energetic flow within the body is said to begin with the Arm Great Yin Lung Channel with a newborn baby's first breath. It moves in an ordered flow through each of the channels, ending with Leg Absolute Yin Liver Channel, which then moves back into Lung, thus starting the process all over again. As you read the pathways of the channels, you might note that where one channel ends, the next channel along this cycle begins. This Cycle of Tides takes place within a 24-hour period of time. It ceases only when life ceases. The order of placement of the channels and points below reflects their relative position within this cycle.

The descriptions of each organ and channel here will help to give you an idea of their placement within the body and the range of influence that each has. Each of the channel pathways include both superficial and internal branches. The internal branches pass through organs and other structures such as the diaphragm. Superficial branches lie on the surface of the body. It is on these superficial branches that acupoints can be found.

In these descriptions I have differentiated between the organ, the channel (the pathway for the movement of energy), and the energy associated with both. The name of the organ channel and the energy associated with that channel are capitalized (as in Lung); lower case is used to refer to the organ itself (lung). Hopefully these simple descriptions of the meridians and their related tissues and energies will help give you a sense of why we treat the arm to support the lungs, or why treating the lower legs might be useful in helping your little one to recover from a bout of diarrhea.

Arm Great Yin Lung

As mentioned previously, the body's flow of qi is said to begin with the Arm Great Yin Lung channel. Lung is considered to be the "tender organ" because it is the one that is most adversely affected by negative substances or energies: air pollution, cold weather or temperatures, and viruses, for example. Of all the organs, the lungs alone come into direct contact with the environment via the breathing passages. The internal environment (the alveoli within the lung) interfaces with the external environment (the air that has been breathed in) in the lungs.

The lungs administer respiration, are in control of qi and air, and have a role in the movement of water within the body. The surface of the body—the skin, hair, and pores—is ruled by Lung energy. It controls sweat and aids in detoxifying the body and maintaining body temperature. The nose is the sense organ that is related to Lung.

Diseases affecting the chest, throat, nose, and lungs come under the domain of Lung.

The Arm Great Yin Lung channel begins in the middle warmer,* between the navel and the breastbone. It moves deep into the torso to encircle the transverse colon. It then ascends through the diaphragm before entering into the lungs. It continues to move upward toward the throat and then crosses the upper chest to arrive at the surface of the body at the deltopectoral groove, the place where the torso meets the upper arm. From there it moves down the outer part of the front of the arm, forearm, wrist, and thumb to end at the nail bed of the thumb.

There are nine points on the Lung channel.

Arm Great Yin Lung is paired with the Arm Bright Yang Colon.

---

*For an explanation of the warmers, see page 36.

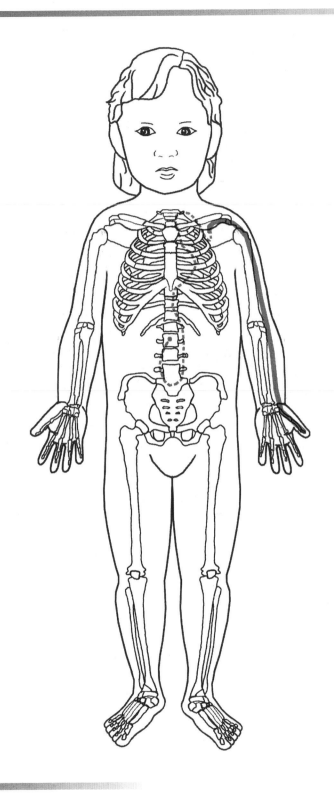

The Arm Great Yin
Lung channel

Arm Bright Yang Colon

The function of the colon is to salvage water from the fecal matter that is passed on to it by the small intestine. Like the lungs, the colon is involved with water metabolism.

The Arm Bright Yang Colon channel begins on the thumb side of the nail bed of the index finger. It passes up through the index finger to the back of the outer side of the wrist, forearm, and arm. It enters into the torso at the edge of the shoulder. It crosses the upper back and passes through the shoulder where it branches, one branch moving internally to pass through the lung and the diaphragm on its way to the colon. From the colon that branch continues to descend to the side of the lower leg below the knee. The other branch remains on the surface, passing up through the neck, crossing the cheek, and curving around the lip to end beside the flare of the nostril on the opposite side of the nose. From here a deep branch enters into the lower gum.

There are twenty points on the Colon channel.

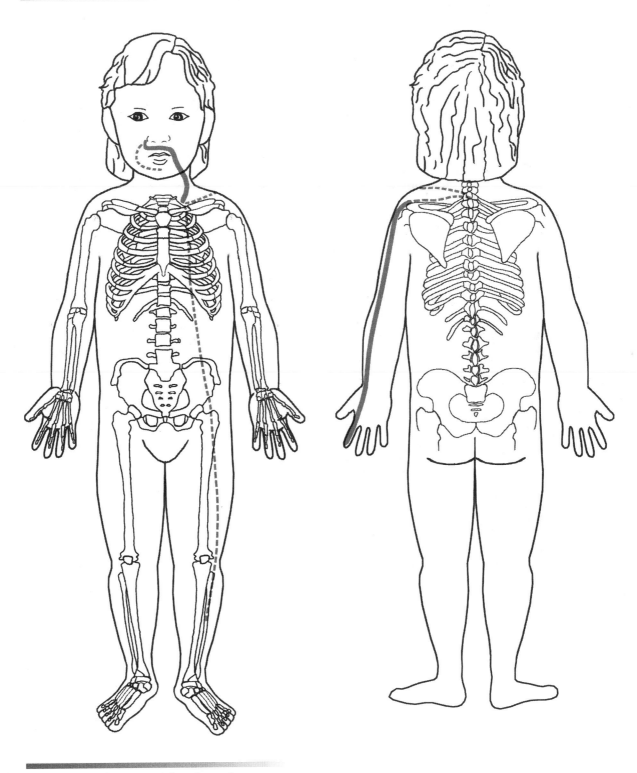

The Arm Bright Yang Colon channel
shown from the front and back

Leg Bright Yang Stomach

The function of the stomach is to receive and digest food before moving it to the small intestine for further processing.

The Leg Bright Yang Stomach channel begins at the flare of the nostril, where the Colon channel ends. It moves up the side of the nose before it emerges just beneath the eye. It passes down over the cheek, around the mouth, and across the jaw. One branch continues to the angle of the jaw and then moves upward to end at the upper hairline. Another branch descends to the top of the clavicle where it passes through to the back before it moves down into the torso. It descends through the diaphragm, and through the stomach, spleen, and large intestine, to emerge at the end of the pubic bone. A superficial branch, running parallel to the internal branch, moves downward from the upper chest to the lower abdomen. The two branches merge at the pubic bone before curving to the outer part of the front of the thigh. The channel runs down the outer part of the front of the thigh and lower leg, passes over the top of the foot and ends at the second toe.

There are forty-five points on the Stomach channel.

Leg Bright Yang Stomach is paired with Leg Great Yin Spleen

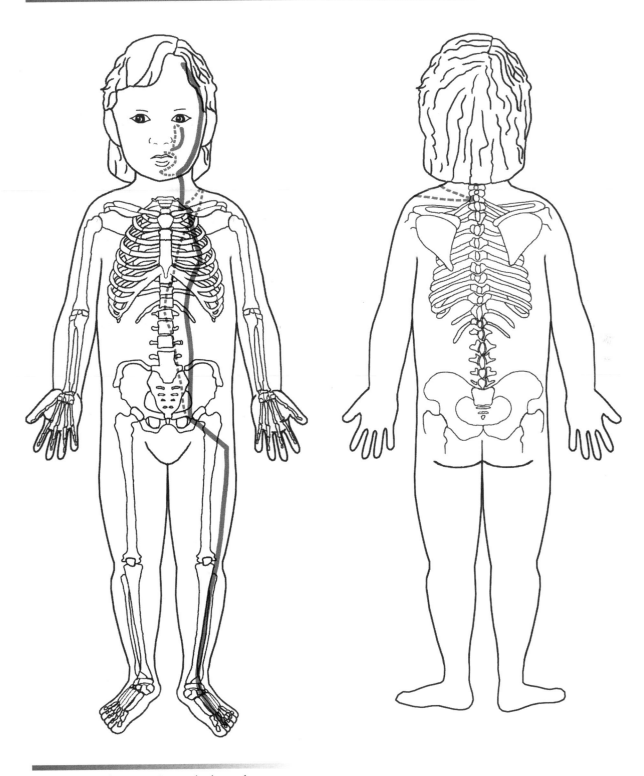

The Leg Bright Yang Stomach channel
shown from the front and back

Leg Great Yin Spleen

Leg Great Yin Spleen is the controller of the digestive function, regulating and balancing the digestive process. The spleen and the stomach together constitute the middle warmer, where digestion takes place. Spleen produces blood, keeps blood in the vessels, and is responsible for keeping the organs in their places; this organ system rules the muscles and limbs. The sense organ associated with Spleen is the mouth.

Digestive disorders or dysfunction, some menstrual disorders, and problems associated with the muscular fatigue and weakness are under the domain of Spleen.

The Leg Great Yin Spleen channel begins at the inner nail bed of the big toe. It moves along the big toe and arch before crossing the ankle in front of the anklebone. It ascends the inside of the lower leg and thigh to the torso. The channel enters into the torso to move through the spleen and stomach organs, then passes through the diaphragm and disperses into the heart. A branch moves up the surface of the torso from the thigh to the upper chest and then to the side of the body, where it ends. From the chest, a deep branch ascends to connect to the tongue.

There are twenty-one points on the Spleen channel.

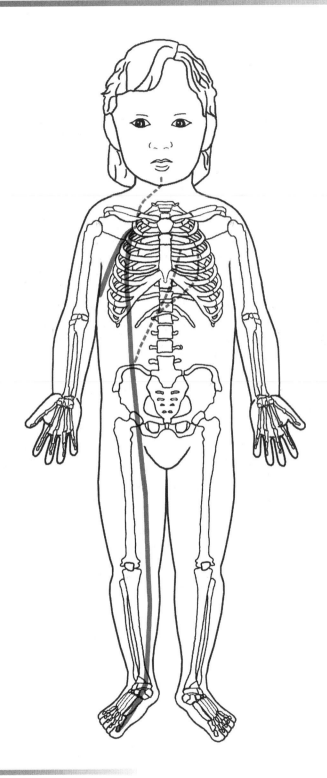

The Leg Great Yin Spleen channel

Arm Lesser Yin Heart

Arm Lesser Yin Heart governs blood. It controls the blood vessels and has fundamental responsibility for the movement of the blood within the vessels. It is said to "house the mind," meaning that mental and emotional activity, thought, memory, sleep, and consciousness are governed by Heart. The tongue is the sense organ associated with Heart.

Pain and fullness in the upper chest and ribs, mental disorders, irritability, shortness of breath, headache, and dizziness are some of the dysfunctions that fall under the domain of Heart.

The Arm Lesser Yin Heart channel begins in the heart. From here it splits into three branches. One branch descends through the diaphragm to connect with the small intestine. One branch ascends to the face, where it joins tissues surrounding the eyes. The third branch travels to the lungs and then emerges at the armpit. From here it descends the front side of the inner arm, forearm, wrist, and palm of the hand, where it passes to the pinky and ends at the inside edge of its nail bed.

There are nine points on the Heart channel.

Arm Lesser Yin Heart is paired with Arm Great Yang Small Intestine

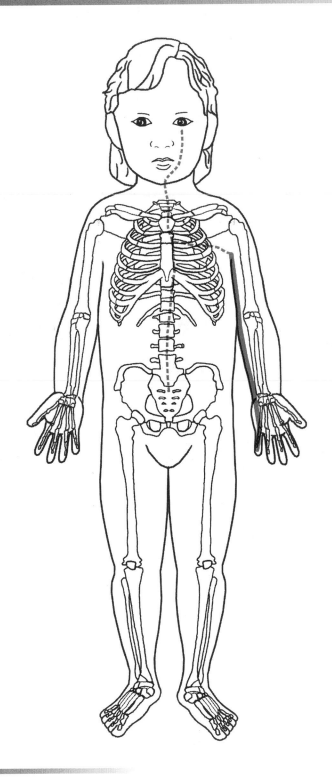

The Arm Lesser Yin Heart channel

Arm Great Yang Small Intestine

The small intestine separates essential nutrients in foods from waste. It passes nutrients into the bloodstream and waste into the large intestine for elimination.

The Arm Great Yang Small Intestine channel begins at the outer edge of the nail bed of the pinky finger. It moves along the edge of the back of the pinky and hand and the inner edge of the back of the forearm to the upper back at the shoulder joint. It passes into the center of the shoulder blade and then up to the top of the shoulder. It moves internally at the base of the neck. It travels to the heart and passes through the diaphragm, then enters into the stomach and the small intestine. The internal branch travels down to the middle of the outer part of the lower leg. From the top of the shoulder a superficial branch passes up over the neck to the cheek, where it travels to the outer edge of the eye and then to the front of the ear.

There are twenty-one points on the Small Intestine channel.

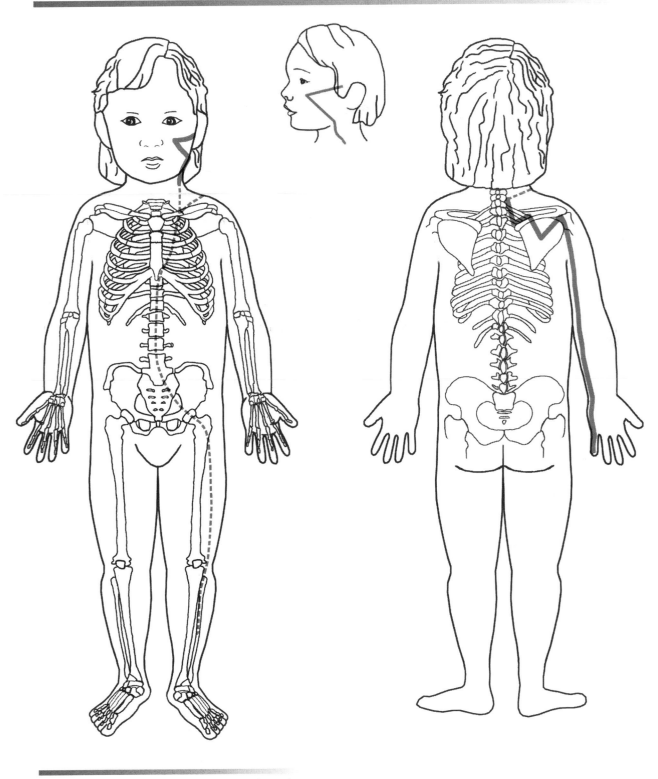

The Arm Great Yang Small Intestine channel
shown from the front, back, and head and
neck profile

Leg Great Yang Bladder

The bladder is responsible for the storage of urine before it is excreted.

The Leg Great Yang Bladder channel begins at the inner corner of the eye. It moves up the forehead and over the head to the base of the skull, where it separates into two parallel superficial branches that descend alongside the spine. When the inner branch reaches the low back it moves into the torso, first into the kidneys and then to the bladder. From there it moves over the buttock, passes over the back of the thigh, and ends at the back of the knee. The outer branch descends alongside the spine and onto the buttock. It connects with the inner branch behind the knee and then descends the back of the calf, around the outer anklebone, to follow along the blade of the foot and end at the outer part of the nail bed of the pinky toe.

There are sixty-seven points on the Bladder channel.

The Bladder points that run alongside the spine have particular clinical significance. They are considered to be especially useful in the treatment of chronic diseases affecting the cardiac, respiratory, gastrointestinal, reproductive, and urinary systems.

Leg Great Yang Bladder is paired with Leg Lesser Yin Kidney

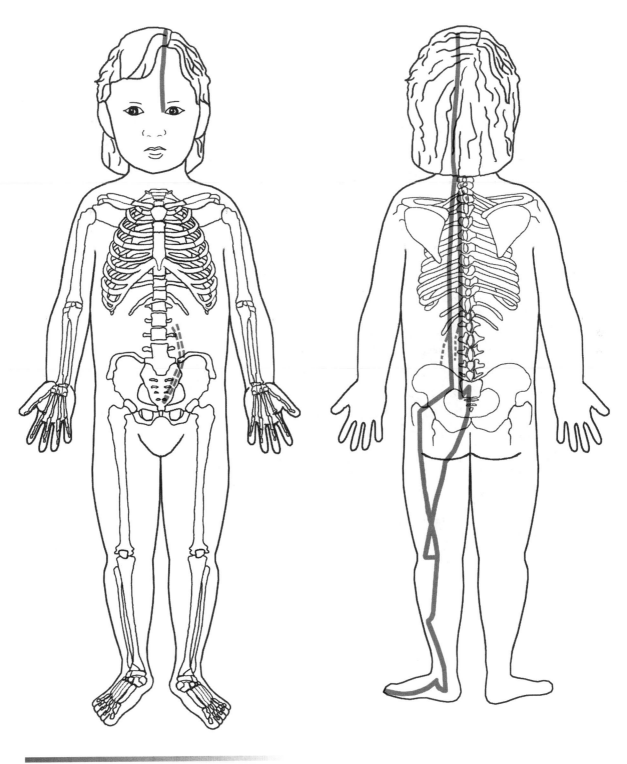

The Leg Great Yang Bladder channel shown
from the front and back

Leg Lesser Yin Kidney

Leg Lesser Yin Kidney is said to contain and store essential substances, specifically the qi that is derived from the parents. Kidney contains the qi that is the driving force for growth, maturity, and reproduction. The solidity of the bones and the nature and quality of the blood and marrow are said to relate to the condition of Kidney. In its cleansing and filtering action, kidney dominates water metabolism. The ear is the sense organ related to Kidney.

Genitourinary disorders, menstrual and reproductive disorders, digestive disorders, abdominal pain, chest pain, respiratory disorders, and dizziness are some of the diverse conditions that fall under the domain of Kidney.

The Leg Lesser Yin Kidney channel begins at the pinky toe. It crosses to the hollow in the sole of the forefoot, easily located when the toes are pointed. It moves to the inside anklebone and then up the inside of the lower leg, knee, and thigh to the base of the spine. It moves up through the lower spine before it enters into the kidneys. Here it separates into two branches. One branch travels up through the liver and the diaphragm, enters into the lungs, moves up through the throat, and ends at the root of the tongue. A branch separates from the lung, connects with the heart, and disperses into the chest. Another branch from the kidney descends to enter into the bladder. From here the channel emerges on the lower abdomen and ascends the front of the torso beside its midline. It ends beside the breastbone, underneath the collarbones.

There are twenty-seven points on the Kidney channel.

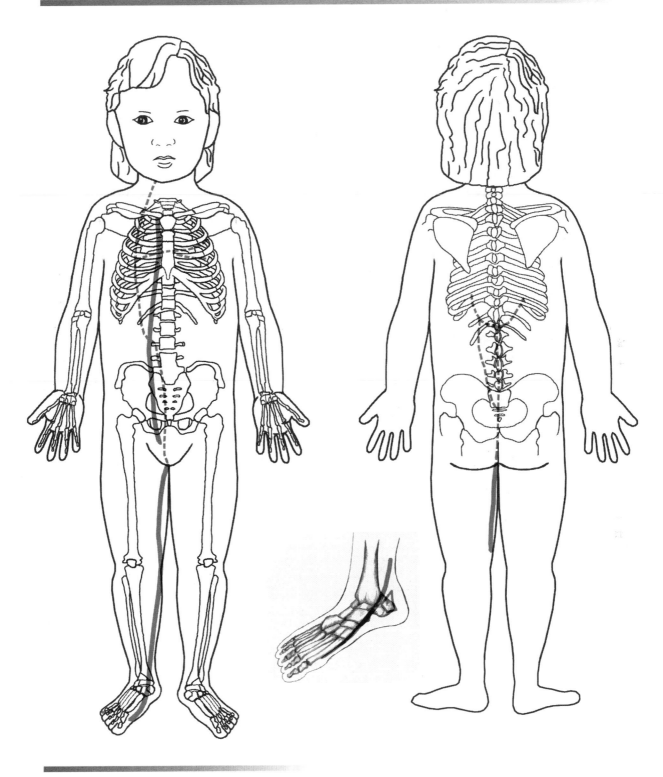

*The Leg Lesser Yin Kidney channel shown from
the front, back, and through the medial foot*

Arm Absolute Yin Pericardium

Arm Absolute Yin Pericardium is considered an external envelope or covering of the heart, and is thus related to Heart. The sphere of influence of Pericardium is the same as that of Heart: it governs blood and mind. The mental and emotional state is considered to be within the domain of Pericardium.

Arm Absolute Yin Pericardium channel begins in the chest. An internal branch descends through the diaphragm and then connects with the upper, middle, and lower warmers. A superficial branch emerges on the chest several inches below the armpit. It then goes up to the armpit before it descends the center of the front of the upper arm, forearm, palm, and middle finger, where it ends beside its nail bed.

There are nine points on the Pericardium channel.

Arm Absolute Yin Pericardium is paired with Arm Lesser Yang Triple Warmer.

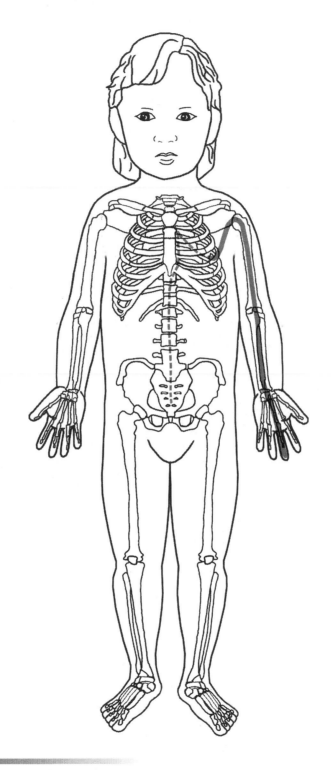

The Arm Absolute Yin Pericardium
channel shown from the front

Arm Lesser Yang Triple Warmer

The Arm Lesser Yang Triple Warmer is considered to represent the functions of digestion, assimilation, and elimination. Traditional Chinese thought describes three "warmers" that are responsible for these functions. The upper warmer is comprised of heart and lungs. The middle warmer is comprised of the stomach and spleen. The lower warmer is comprised of the kidneys, bladder, and intestines. The middle warmer is said to receive substance (food and drink) and break it down, so the upper warmer can disperse its qi throughout the body and the lower warmer can excrete its waste.

The Arm Lesser Yang Triple Warmer channel begins on the nail bed of the ring finger. It moves up the back of the hand, forearm, and upper arm to the shoulder and upper back. From here an internal branch moves to the center of the chest. One part of this branch connects with the pericardium before it passes through the diaphragm to the abdomen, where it connects with the upper, middle, and lower warmers. A branch crosses from the upper shoulder up the neck. It passes around the ear and across the temple to the eyebrow.

There are twenty-three points on the Triple Warmer channel.

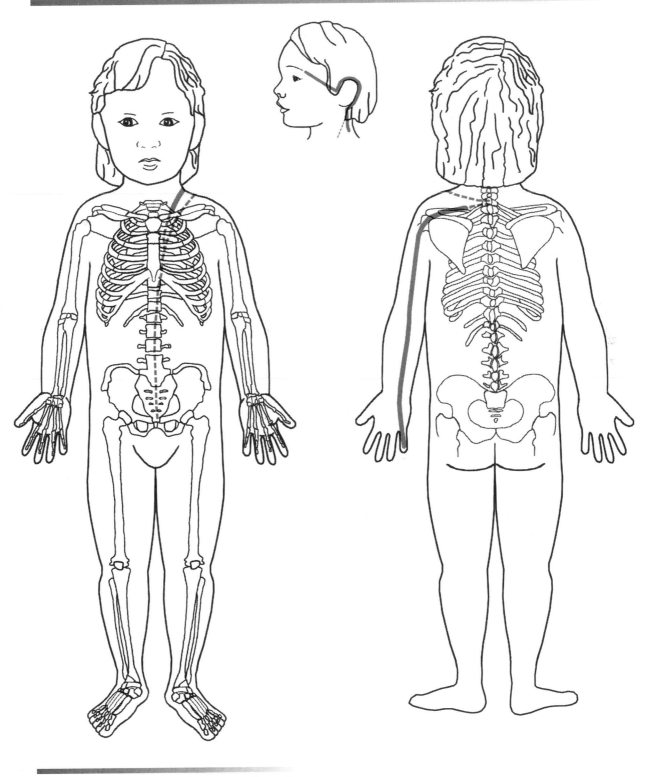

The Arm Lesser Yang Triple Warmer channel shown from the front, back, and head and neck profile

Leg Lesser Yang Gall Bladder

The gall bladder stores and secretes bile.

The Leg Lesser Yang Gall Bladder channel begins at the outside of the eye. It crosses the temple before traveling around the ear. It traverses the head several times before it reaches the upper shoulder. An internal branch crosses the cheek and then enters into the torso, crosses the diaphragm, and connects with the liver and gall bladder. It continues down into the lower torso to encircle the genitals and then emerge at the hip. A superficial branch travels from the upper shoulder to the outer side of the chest, rib cage, and hip, where it meets the internal branch. It continues to descend the outside part of the thigh, knee, lower leg, and ankle. It crosses the top of the foot between the fourth and fifth toes, ending at the nail bed of the fourth toe.

There are forty-four points on the Gall Bladder channel.

Leg Lesser Yang Gall Bladder is paired with Leg Absolute Yin Liver.

The Leg Lesser Yang Gall Bladder channel shown in the head and neck

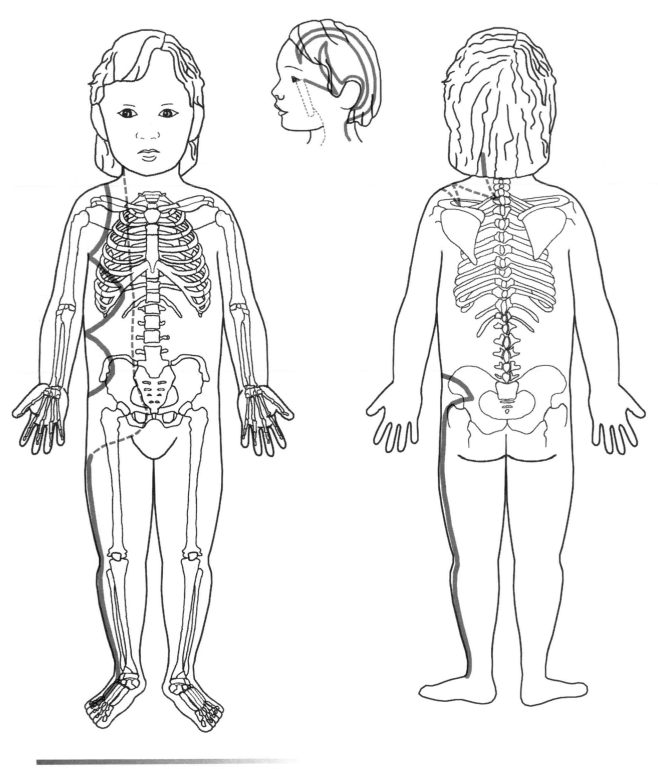

*The Leg Lesser Yang Gall Bladder channel
shown from the front, back, and head and
neck profile*

Leg Absolute Yin Liver

Leg Absolute Yin Liver is responsible for several important functions. Its first function is the smooth flowing of qi throughout the body. Emotions play an important part in this. There is a relationship between constrained or restricted Liver energy and emotional tension characterized by anger, frustration, rage, and depression. If you consider how your body gets locked up during emotionally charged times, you can begin to understand how the flow of qi is impaired; everything is impaired—muscles, digestion, circulation. Proper functioning of the liver is important for digestion and the unimpeded flow of bile. Liver regulates the volume of circulating blood. It is in control of the tendons and affects the ability to move and take part in physical activity. The sense organ associated with Liver is the eye.

Gynecological dysfunction and diseases, menstrual disorders, digestive disorders, muscle spasms, and cramps are under the domain of Liver.

The Leg Absolute Yin Liver channel begins at the nail bed of the big toe. It crosses the top of the foot between the big toe and the second toe, crosses the ankle, and travels up the inside of the lower leg and thigh to the groin. It encircles the genitals before entering into the lower belly. Internally it moves upward and enters into the liver and gall bladder. It travels up through the diaphragm to the lungs and then through the back of the throat to connect with the tissues around the eyes. It continues up the forehead to the top of the head. A superficial branch crosses the lower abdomen to the bottom of the ribs before continuing up to its end at the rib cage.

There are fourteen points on the Liver channel.

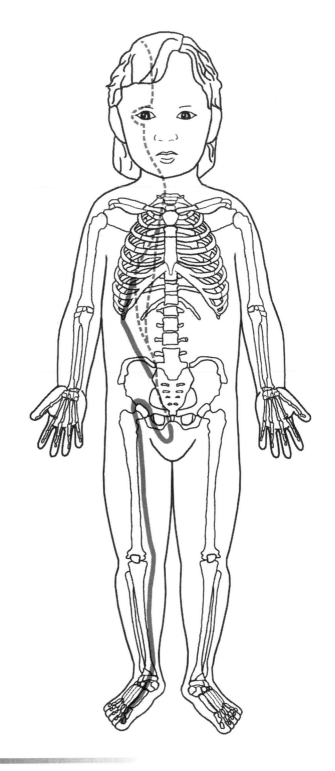

The Leg Absolute Yin Liver channel
shown from the front

The Extraordinary Vessels: Conception Vessel and Governing Vessel

Although they are not organ channels, these two Extraordinary Vessels need to be mentioned because of their significance and use.

The Conception Vessel is the sea of the yin channels. It is considered to have a regulating effect on all yin channels.

The Conception Vessel travels along the midline of the front of the body. It begins in the lower abdomen and emerges in the perineum. It runs up the front of the body and throat. Its superficial path ends underneath the lips. Internally it curves around the mouth and ends underneath the eyes.

There are twenty-four points on Conception Vessel.

Governing Vessel is the sea of the yang channels. It is considered to have a regulating effect on all yang channels.

Governing Vessel has four pathways. Its superficial pathway begins in the lower abdomen. It emerges in the perineum and then runs up the back of the body and neck. It travels over the back and top of the head, down over the forehead, and ends just underneath the nose.

There are twenty-eight points on Governing Vessel.

These are generalized descriptions of only fourteen of the fifty-nine channels within the system. Hopefully these descriptions give you a glimpse into the complexity of the movement of qi, and will give you an idea of how each pathway intersects with two or more organs within the body. Missing from these descriptions is the vast number of intersections that exist among each of the pathways.

Think about these relationships and connections as you touch your child. Think about what you want to accomplish with the treatment you are giving your child. Touch her with curiosity. Touch her with an open mind. Listen to what is happening under your hands. You may feel areas of warmth, coolness, fullness, hollowness. Work on and around them and see what happens. The results may surprise and please you. You might just encounter the wonder of the body healing itself.

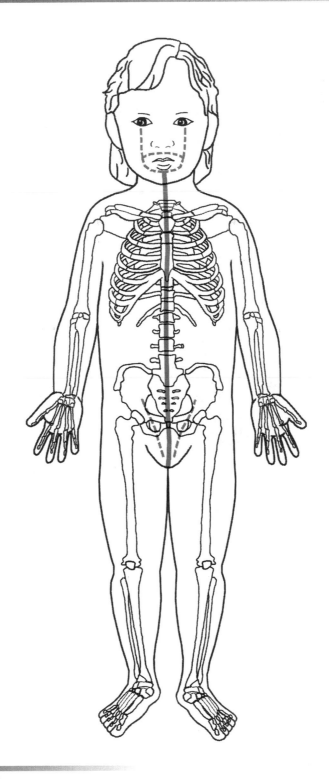

The Conception Vessel

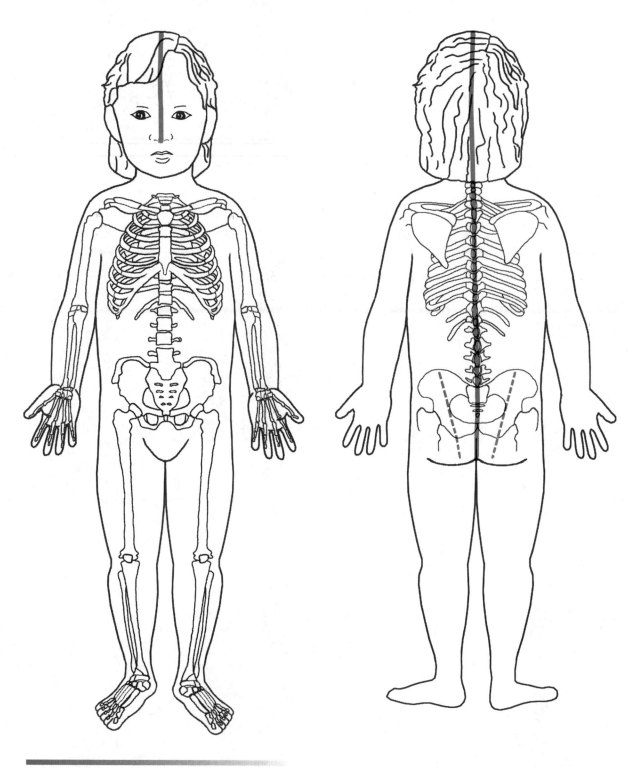

The Governing Vessel shown from the front and back.

PART II
TREATMENTS

Maintaining Good Health

What is it?

You know a healthy child when you see one. You see a normal, energetic, happy, impish little one enjoying life. You can see a glint in the clear eyes of a healthy child. She has enough energy to move continuously. Her digestion is good—foods go in with ease and come out just as easily. She sleeps well, and she awakens fully ready to start the day. When she's running and playing there is no hint of breathing problems—her nose isn't running or congested, she doesn't cough, and she's never out of breath. Her skin is clear and her complexion radiant. Nothing hurts. She has no complaints. And all you want to do is keep it that way!

What causes it?

Youth. And a good diet, reasonable exercise, and sufficient rest.

How can you help?

We have to be vigilant these days. It is unfortunately the case that environmental and social issues exist that may hinder our efforts to be healthy.

Years back, you could go outside and drink the water from the local stream and eat the vegetables you grew in your yard. You knew they were good: the stream was pure and the vegetables fresh. But the world in which we live today is not like that anymore. Residues of plastics, cosmetics, pesticides, insecticides, artificial hormones, pharmaceuticals, disinfectants, and other synthetic materials can be found in the water supplies, the air that we breathe, and the soils that surround our homes. Chemical contaminants can be found in the products we use around our homes, on our bodies, and in the materials from which our homes have been constructed. We are continuously exposed to these substances at a very low level. As they have been found on the earth upon which we live, they have been found circulating within our bodies. Some of them have been found to be toxic, and yet there is little information on their long-term effects on our health. I believe that it is wise to try and limit our exposure to them.

You can help to reduce exposure to *chemical contaminants* in and around your home in the following ways.

- Keep kids away from solvents: paints, non-water based glues, furniture strippers, gasoline, perfumes, nail polish, and nail polish remover. If you must use these products, make sure the area is well ventilated when you do so.
- Keep your kids out of the house or yard when you are using insecticides or pesticides.
- Make sure you read labels on household cleaning supplies—and follow the directions for safe use.
- Air out your dry-cleaned clothing before bringing it home, and take dry-cleaned clothes out of the plastic bags once they are in your home.
- Avoid using plastic wraps and containers to store food or water, and don't use them to heat foods in the microwave or to store hot foods.
- Limit your use of plastic bottled water. An in-home reverse osmosis or filtration system or a filter pitcher will adequately purify your water and limit your exposure to contaminants leached from plastic bottles.
- Avoid using the clear plastic baby bottles or cups that are made of polycarbonate plastic.
- Replace any old plastic containers or bottles that are scratched.
- Avoid the use of non-stick cookware. If your non-stick cookware begins to scratch, replace it.

Educate yourself on the problem of household contaminants—it is one that is here to stay. We can try to minimize our exposure, but we won't eliminate it in our lifetime. You don't have to be crazed or fanatical about it—but you can be aware. Awareness will, in and of itself, lead you to exercising greater caution for yourself and your family regarding chemical contaminants.

Do we really need anti-bacterial cleansers?

In the last decade it has become increasingly clear that our excessive use of anti-biotics in humans and in the animals used for our food supplies has led to more and more powerful bacteria that have grown resistant to the antibiotics we have at hand. Some have even become resistant to the most powerful antibiotics that have so far been developed.

The use of anti-microbial (so-called anti-bacterial) soaps and cleaning supplies in our homes, particularly those containing triclosan, has exacerbated this problem. Look around your kitchen and bathroom. Do you use anti-bacterial soaps and cleansers? You really don't need them.

There are many products on the market made from naturally occurring cleaning substances. A vinegar and water solution will do the job of cleaning your kitchen and bathroom very well. Baking soda is a great abrasive cleaner. Even a dilute bleach solution is a relatively benign alternative. Try some of these. They work and they won't add to the problem of antibiotic-resistant organisms.

The social issue is probably somewhat easier to deal with. It's one about which we have far greater control. Obesity and diabetes are rapidly becoming the most common chronic childhood conditions. The situation is approaching epidemic proportions. Kids are becoming overweight due to poor eating habits and lack of exercise. More and more overweight children are being diagnosed with high cholesterol and high blood pressure, and when a child is obese he is at a greater risk for developing diabetes and/or cardiovascular disease as an adult. You can help your kids by watching what they eat and what they do. Teaching your kids about the basics of a healthful diet and the need for regular exercise is an important way you can help them stay healthy as children and grow into healthy adults.

The foods we take in are so important for all of us because it is literally the components of our foods that make up the components of our bodies. Consider this—my body is made up of the same stuff that this earth is made of, by some force far greater than me. So how should I nourish my body? With man-made stuff? Or with the stuff that comes forth from Mother Earth naturally?

My personal preference is for foods as nature intended them to be. I believe that if you can't pronounce an ingredient you should think twice before eating it; and you should think hard before giving it to your child—whose body is growing and developing. Choose whole, natural foods, foods that are organic are not produced with chemical fertilizers, antibiotics, hormones, or growth modifiers; they do not contain genetically modified organisms (GMOs), chemicals, preservatives or additives, colorings or other artificial additives; they are not distorted or transformed by any means. Organic foods are more easily obtained these days. To the extent that you can, try to include them in your diet.

- Feed your kids (and yourselves) a well-balanced, varied diet.
- Complete proteins such as lean cuts of beef and pork, poultry, fish, eggs, and low fat dairy products are important for tissue development. Eating lean cuts of meat allows you to keep your consumption of animal fats to a minimum. This will limit your intake of both saturated fats, which contribute to obesity and heart disease, and the antibiotic and hormone residues that are stored in the fats. Naturally or organically produced meats, poultry, eggs, and dairy are grown both humanely and without the use of antibiotics and hormones. They are a good choice if you can find them.
- Beans, soy, nuts, and whole grains are good vegetable sources of protein and are a beneficial component of a healthy diet.
- Choose organic fruits and vegetables that are locally produced in season. Avoid fruits and vegetables that are grown outside of this country. Be aware that foods that are imported from other countries may not follow the same pesticide regulations that are in place in the United States. To avoid exposure to these pesticides and their residues, you would have to avoid fruits and vegetables

that are out of season. Knowing that cantaloupe, honeydew, and watermelon aren't harvested in January in the United States, I don't purchase them when I see them in the produce section of the grocery store.

- Eat a diet that includes whole grains and whole grain products: wheat, oats, brown rice, barley, quinoa. Products that are made from organic ingredients and do not contain chemical additives and preservatives are preferable.

- If you choose to eat sweets, use moderate amounts of naturally occurring raw or turbinado sugar, maple syrup, or honey in your foods rather than using artificial sweeteners and foods and drinks that contain them.

- Limit your consumption of refined carbohydrates, white flour, and white sugar products. Some foods really should be occasional treats: cookies, pastries, candy, ice cream, sugared drinks such as iced teas, sodas, and drink mixes. Many of these foods are high in calories and have little nutrient value. They fill you up without providing substantive value to the body. Soft drinks are particularly deceiving. The average 12-ounce serving of soda contains approximately 10 teaspoons of sugar.

- Try to limit your consumption of fast foods, fried foods, and junk foods. Between the questionable nutritional quality and the high amounts of salt and saturated fats, you'll be doing yourself and your kids a favor if you make these foods very occasional treats, rather than weekly fare.

- Avoid the use of prepackaged, prepared foods and foods that contain preservatives and chemical additives. It's so important to read food labels. If you can't pronounce an ingredient, it's likely that it's an artificial additive.

- Encourage your children to drink purified water and diluted fruit juices. Babies and young children should be limited to drinking no more than 4 to 6 ounces of fruit juice daily. Fruit juices are often high in sugars. When kids fill up on juices they often don't have room left over for more nutritious foods.

- In my mind the use of purified water is becoming more and more important. In past years, hormone residues from livestock excrement and traces of prescription drugs from human use have been found in the waterways. We really don't know about the purity of our drinking supply. Perhaps we are better off being cautious now, rather than sorry years from now.

It's also important to teach your children good eating habits—not just what they eat, but how and when they eat it. It is said that the most important meal of the day is breakfast. A breakfast that is rich in whole grains and proteins will provide the fuel that you and your child need to make it through the long morning with enough energy to think clearly and function well. Sugary cereals and pastries provide an energy surge that is quickly followed with a period of fatigue—the result of blood sugar highs and lows.

Encourage your children to have their meals and snacks seated at the table, rather than in front of a television, alone in their room, walking around the house or as they rush out the door.

Eat together and share your enjoyment of good food with your children. Healthful meals, eaten together, can become a pleasurable time to connect as a family, to converse about the day, sharing experiences.

If you expose your children to many different types of foods, they will experience the pleasure of fine food early on in life. If you teach them to eat well early on, they will eat well for a lifetime. (Notwithstanding the deviation that will undoubtedly take place during their teens and twenties. So be it—they'll return.)

These guidelines for healthful eating may sound daunting. They really aren't. If you've already begun to alter your diet and your kids' diets, that's great—keep it up. If you're just beginning, take one aspect at a time so you don't become overwhelmed with it all. Start with increasing their fruits and vegetables and limit their refined carbohydrates (white sugar and white flour). Over time, slowly change the way you approach the grocery store. Read labels. Be patient. If you keep at it, over time you will see a change in your family's health.

Exercise is an important part of keeping healthy; it's good for your body and it's good for your mind. Some of us, including our kids, spend way too much time working and playing on a computer, watching television, and playing video games. It's hard enough to be an adult with a sedentary lifestyle. Kids have so much energy that needs to be expended. They never sit still. Can you imagine being a kid who can't run around during the day because of the demands placed on him by school? It isn't all that uncommon! All that pent-up energy—what do they do with it? Encourage your kids to get outside and move—hike, walk, ride a bike, dance, play ball. Do it with them! When they see that you are exercising and taking care of your health, they will follow along.

Sleep is an important part of keeping the body healthy and the mind sharp. Make sure your kids get enough rest and sleep. Most kids need about 10 hours of sleep a night. Encourage your kids to go to bed at an hour that allows them sufficient sleep to meet their individual needs. A bedtime routine is a peaceful bonding time that can start as early as infancy. Reading together, talking, singing, hugs and kisses promote a sense of calm connectedness that is good for both you and your child. If your child isn't ready for sleep, set the stage for him to take some time to wind down: read or listen to music together. I believe that television and video games are best avoided before bed. They arouse rather than calm. The routine, the rest, and the sleep will help keep your children healthy, happy, and alert.

The simplest way to avoid getting sick is to practice good hygiene. Teach your kids about the importance of bathing daily and brushing their teeth. Make sure to wash your hands regularly and teach your children to wash theirs. A thorough 15-second wash of the hands with soap and water or the use of an alcohol based hand rub is the easiest way to prevent the spread of disease.

Eating well, moving your body, sleeping well and practicing good hygiene: It is an elixir for good health—for all of us.

Treatment

A treatment for general health can be done at any time: after a bath, before bed, any time you're both calm. This treatment will help to relax the muscles, increase circulation, stimulate digestion, and calm the mind.

All of the shaded areas in the treatment illustrations are useful in keeping your child strong and healthy. Some areas are shaded lightly, others somewhat darker. The lightly shaded areas need the least amount of work; the darkest areas need the most attention. Work on the lightly shaded areas just once or twice during the course of the treatment; work on the darker areas more frequently, staying at each area no more than 3 to 5 seconds at a time. When you treat an older child, adolescent, or adult, you can locate the acupoints within the darkly shaded areas. But when you treat a baby or young child, working generally in the area of an acupoint will produce the desired result.

Use a gentle touch when you massage your child. When you are working on a baby, all the pressure that's needed is the degree of pressure you would use if you were finger painting or checking to see if a cake is finished baking.

Take your time; relax. This can be fun and pleasurable for both of you.

1. Start with a massage of the forehead. Stroke from the bridge of the nose up toward the hairline, and then from the midpoint of the forehead out toward the temples.

    Long, calming strokes set the stage for the relaxation of the whole body.

2. Gently massage the neck, beginning just underneath the ears and working down toward the collarbones.

    Treatment here will release the sternocleidomastoid (SCM) and scalene muscles and help to promote the free flow oe lymphatic fluid into the upper torso.

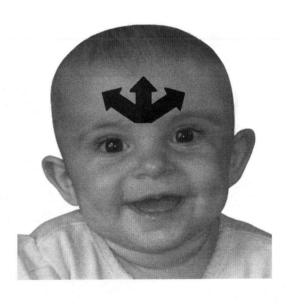

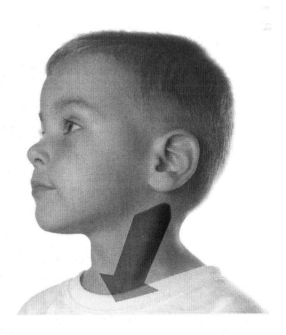

Treatment areas on the face and neck for maintaining good health

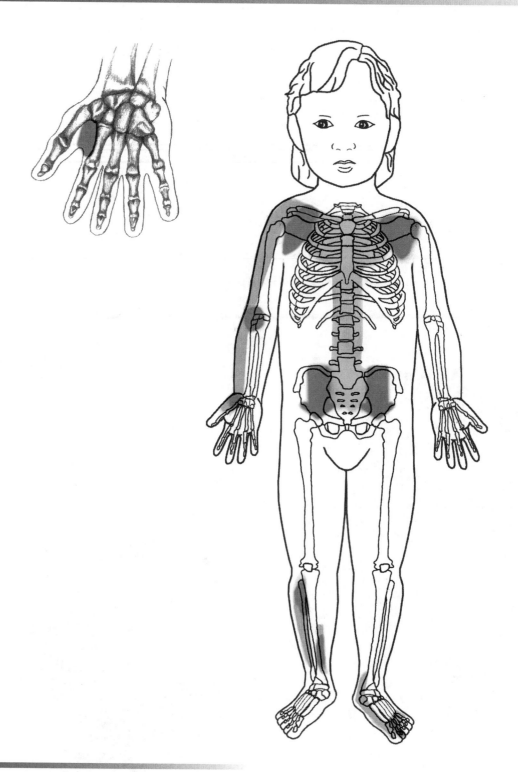

Treatment areas on the body and hand for
maintaining good health

3. Gently massage the center of the chest, beginning at the top of the breastbone and working down toward the belly.

4. Starting at the center of the upper part of the breastbone, massage the upper chest out toward the arms. Spend a bit of time working in the area where the arms meet the body.

   Pectoralis major lies on the upper chest. It tends to tighten both with emotional stresses and respiratory ailments. Keeping the muscles supple will help to release stress and help the lungs to function optimally. Lung 1 and Lung 2, in the deltopectoral groove (the intersection of the deltoid muscle and pectoralis major) support lung function.

5. Massage the outside of the front of the arms from the shoulders toward the thumb. Spend a bit more time at the elbow fold and the fleshy palm side of the thumb.

   Lung 5 and Lung 10 support lung function.

6. Massage the back side of the hand between the thumb and the index finger.

   Colon 4 helps to strengthen the system. Colon 4 works with Liver 3 to calm the system.

7. Massage the lower belly. Work on each side of the belly button, moving down toward the lower belly. (If you keep your palms down, keeping your hands on the belly without losing contact, it will feel less ticklish. Of course, tickling can be fun, too!)

   Massage of the lower abdomen helps maintain healthy bowel function.

8. Massage the outside of the lower leg from just underneath the knee to the ankle. Spend a bit more time just underneath the knee.

   Stomach 36 works with Spleen 6 to help strengthen immune function.

9. Massage the inside of the lower leg a couple of inches above the inner ankle.

   Spleen 6 works with Stomach 36 to help strengthen immune function.

10. Massage the feet, beginning at the inside of the ankle and working down through the arch toward the big toe. Massage in between the long bones of the feet, focusing more attention between the long bones of the big toe and the second toe.

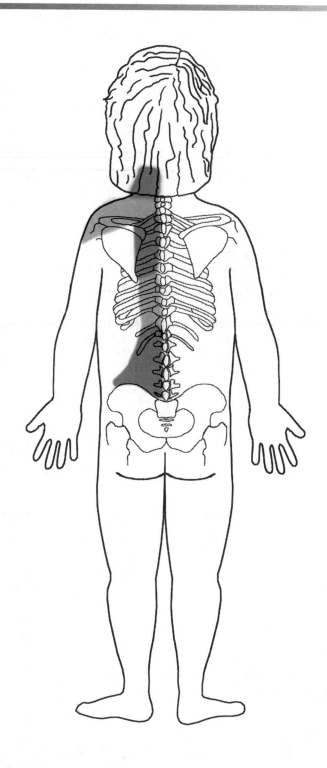

Treatment areas for maintaining good health—along the back

Aspects of digestion, assimilation, and elimination will be stimulated with the massage of the Spleen and Kidney channels on the medial foot. Liver 3 works with Colon 4 to calm the system.

11. Massage the tops of the shoulders, working from where the neck meets the body to the outer edge of the shoulders.

    Upper trapezius is the muscle that most easily develops restrictions and trigger points. Massaging this muscle will help to nip any restrictions in the bud. Each of the yang meridians travels through this area. Their release contributes to the free flow of energy through the system.

12. Massage the back on both sides of the spine, spending a good deal of time in the areas just between the shoulder blades and just above the pelvis.

    Working on the erector spinae muscles helps to release tension and stress, both physical and emotional. The Bladder points alongside the spine affect cardiovascular and respiratory function, digestion, assimilation, elimination, and urinary function.

13. Finish with long strokes gently massaging the muscles lying beside the spine, beginning at the upper back and stroking down toward the pelvis.

    Soothing strokes just feel good and are incredibly calming!

Common Cold

When should you check with your doctor?

Most of the time, a cold will come and go without any need to consult a physician. However, if you believe that your child has developed an infection, such as sinusitis, an ear infection, or bronchitis, you should consult with your doctor. Check in with your doctor if this is your baby's first cold, if he has a fever of 100.4° F and is three months old or younger, or if the baby is older than four months and has a fever that is higher than 102° F. If your child has a non-stop cough or a cough that lasts longer than two weeks, if she coughs up thick mucus, has asthmatic wheezing, or has difficulty breathing, call your doctor. If she develops a rash, has an earache or stomachache, or can't swallow or urinate without pain, consult with your doctor.

What is it?

A cold is an upper respiratory infection (URI). Upper respiratory infection is one of the most common illnesses, and, in the long run, one of the least harmful. It's estimated that most adults have two to four colds a year, and most children have many more than that. In their earliest years, when the immune system is developing, children can have as many as eight to ten colds a year, particularly those children who attend childcare or school. Upper respiratory infection is one of the five most common illnesses that keep kids from going to school (along with gastroenteritis, better known as stomach flu; ear infections; conjunctivitis; and sore throat). The number of colds that kids experience each year generally begins to decrease by the time they are six years old.

A cold is a mild inflammation of the membranes lining the nose and throat. It usually lasts from seven to ten days and it will generally resolve on its own. While a cold is typically harmless, it is nonetheless uncomfortable. We've all had them so we know the symptoms and how they make us feel: the runny or stuffed nose, a sore throat, sneezing, coughing, runny eyes, post nasal drip, head congestion and the headache and mild fatigue that goes with it, and possibly a low-grade fever—lower than 101° F. We don't feel terrible, but we don't feel good. We want to sleep, but lying down makes it harder to breath through our nose; sometimes we sneeze or cough more when we're trying to sleep.

Customarily, a cold incubates for about four days. The first three days after a cold has "blossomed" is its most contagious time, when the nasal mucus is clear and very runny. As the cold runs its course, nasal mucus will become thicker and yellow or green in color. This is a good sign; the body is fighting the infection, and the virus is no longer contagious.

While a cold generally runs its course with little or no intervention, it may lead to an ear infection, particularly in an infant or young child (see p. x[**X-ref**]) or a sinus infection in an older child (see p. x [**X-Ref**]).

When is it the flu (influenza) and not a cold?

The symptoms of a cold are similar to that of the flu—but with the flu those symptoms are significantly worse. The symptoms of the flu come on very suddenly. Unlike a cold, with the flu the fever will be high—often higher than 102° F—and it will last for three to four days. There will be body aches, headache, and chills, loss of appetite, and the need to sleep due to extreme fatigue. There may also be runny nose, sneezing, head congestion, and a dry cough that may turn into a bad cough. While the fever and discomfort from the flu usually last for only three or four days, the fatigue and the cough may linger for up to two weeks.

If you believe that your child actually has the flu rather than a cold, talk to your doctor.

What causes it?

A cold is caused by numerous viruses, most commonly the *rhinovirus*, which is highly contagious. Colds are most often spread through tiny droplets of mucus or saliva that are sprayed through the air when you sneeze, cough, or speak. Hand-to-hand contact also can spread the virus. If a child touches his face and then touches a toy—or any object at all—that object can become the source of infection for the next person who touches it. If a sick child touches his face, nose, or mouth and then you touch the child's hands, you can end up with a cold.

How you can help . . .

. . . keep him comfortable

For something that you can do little about, there is quite a bit that you can do to help!

If your infant or baby has a runny nose or crusty dry mucus, you can use a nasal aspirator (a soft nasal suction bulb) to clear the mucus from his nose.

You can help a baby or child with a stuffy nose by placing a couple of drops of additive-free nasal saline (salt water solution) into his nose two or three times a day. Use 1–2 drops in each nostril for a baby and 3–4 drops in each nostril for an older child. Wait a few minutes to allow the saline to loosen the dried mucus, then use a nasal aspirator to clear your baby's nose or have your child blow his nose gently.

For older children, using nasal saline sprays that are specially formulated for children and are free of additives and preservatives is a helpful way to keep mucus moist and moving.

If your child's stuffy nose is keeping him from sleeping, place a humidifier or vaporizer in his room to help keep his mucous membranes from drying out. Dry air in heated homes during winter months dries out the airways and leads to thicker, stickier mucus. The vaporizer or humidifier will moisten the air, soothe dry mucous membranes, thin out thickened mucus, and make breathing easier. If you do use a humidifier or vaporizer, make sure you clean it regularly according to manufacturer directions.

Placing a couple of drops of eucalyptus oil near (not on) his pillow will help open a stuffy nose and make breathing easier.

Keep your child home from childcare or school if you think he is in a contagious phase of a cold, if he has any fever at all (even a low-grade fever), or if he is fatigued or "off" and seems to be coming down with something. A day or two at home might prevent your child from getting sicker and from sharing his cold with others. If your child is older and has many after-school activities, allow him to skip them while he is recovering from a cold as well.

If you are allowing the child to stay home from school, keep him in an area where the temperature is warm and stable. And let him rest. Rest and sleep are the greatest healers. The body knows it. Use that wisdom to your advantage.

If your child is particularly uncomfortable or has a fever, speak to your doctor about giving him acetaminophen (Tylenol) or ibuprofen (Advil). Avoid using aspirin with children. It may cause Reye's syndrome, a rare but potentially harmful disease.

Do cold preparations help?

It has become increasingly clear that antibiotics don't speed the healing of a cold or virus; neither do antihistamines, decongestants, or cough suppressants. Over-the-counter medications may temporarily make us more comfortable, but they do nothing to decrease the time it takes for the body to go through the healing process.

Today there are several over-the-counter preparations that are designed to treat many cold symptoms. Choosing one of these "multi-symptom" preparations can be complex and confusing. Perhaps your child only has one symptom that's making her uncomfortable. Maybe she can't sleep because of a stuffy nose. She may not need the different medications that are in a multi-symptom preparation. Why give her something that she doesn't need? If your child is very uncomfortable and you feel she needs something to help her, try to choose a medicine that is aimed at relieving only the symptom that she's suffering with, and follow the dosage recommendations carefully. That will go a long way toward not over-medicating her.

Over-the-counter preparations are not harmless. Most should not be used for babies and children younger than two years old. They need to be used with caution. If you believe that your baby needs relief from her symptoms or if you are unsure of the cold preparation or dosage that would benefit your older child, speak to your health care provider.

Also, it's important to remember this great truth of how the body works: each symptom has a purpose. Our runny nose is the body clearing the mucous membranes and our cough is moving mucus out of the respiratory tract so we can breathe better. It isn't always best to get rid of every symptom.

. . . prevent him from getting a cold or the flu

In the fall, winter, and early spring, the flu virus is everywhere. So why don't we get colds more often? From the Oriental perspective, if your energy—particularly your *wei chi* (defensive chi)—is strong, your body is easily able to fend off the viruses and bacteria that are all around us all the time. Parents throughout time have warned their children against "getting a draft"—"Put your jacket on, you'll get a cold!" "Keep your head covered." "Don't go out with wet hair— you'll get sick!" Many of us heard these injunctions, or others like them, and probably thought they were nonsense. Well, there's truth in them. Any Oriental medicine practitioner will tell you that the invasion of cold has a negative affect on the body's systems. When it's cold outside, keep your kids warm—keep hats on their heads and socks on their feet, cover their chests, and avoid drafts. Of these, the most important is keeping a hat on their heads—up to 20 percent of your body heat escapes through your head. Something as simple as wearing a baseball cap makes a remarkable difference to total body warmth.

The simplest way to avoid getting sick is to make sure to wash your hands regularly and teach your children to wash theirs. Using soap and warm water or an alcohol-based hand rub (anti-bacterial rubs aren't necessary) is the easiest way to prevent the spread of disease. Colds, the flu, and many other diseases are caused by hand-to-hand contact. Teach your kids to wash after they've touched their face, coughed, or sneezed into their hand or blown their nose if they have a cold. If they don't have a cold, getting one can be prevented if they get into the habit of washing their hands before they eat, after they've used the bathroom, when they come in from playing outdoors, after they've played with or touched the family pet, or after they've been with someone who has a cold. Little things can make the biggest difference.

Teach your children to use tissues to cover their mouth and nose when coughing or sneezing. When tissues are used, make sure to throw them away immediately. If tissues aren't available, teach them to sneeze or cough into the crook of their arm (the bend in their elbow) rather than into their hand. Not only will droplets be prevented from pouring into the air, but there is less of a possibility that they will contaminate objects by touching them with their hands. (If they aren't wearing sleeves, make sure they wash their arms as well as their hands!)

Try to encourage your children to keep their hands, toys, pencils, and anything else that isn't food out of their mouths. Wash toys and other frequently used objects to prevent them from being the source of disease.

Avoid sharing drinking glasses, eating utensils, and towels when someone has a cold. Wash or change drinking glasses (particularly those used in the bathroom) after each use. And be sure to replace his toothbrush after your child has recovered from his cold or flu.

A word on diet

Modifying your child's diet will help him recover from his cold quickly. Dairy products tend to increase the body's mucus production, so avoid giving your sick child any cow's milk or milk products. That includes cheeses, yogurt, cottage cheese, ice cream, and puddings. You can try substituting soy milk and soy-based cheeses.

Fluids help to thin mucus secretions, so make sure he's drinking plenty of liquids. Water, diluted juices, clear broths, and diluted herb teas are good choices. And chicken soup really does do wonders when you have a cold!

Steamed and fresh fruits and vegetables and lightly prepared chicken and fish are easy for your child to digest when he has a cold. Avoid giving your child high fat foods, such as fried foods, fast foods, or processed or fatty meats. They are far more difficult to digest. And as always, keep him away from highly processed foods: white sugar (candy, cookies, pastries, sodas), white flour and bread products, and foods with chemicals and preservatives.

Treatment

Use this treatment to help your little one feel better as his cold runs its course. In many cases you'll find that the cold passes through his system quite quickly after you've treated him one or two times. The aim of this treatment is to open his nasal passages and his chest, ease a sore throat, increase lymphatic drainage, and generally strengthen his system so he can heal quickly.

All of the shaded areas in the treatment illustrations show where to work on your child when he has a cold. Some areas are shaded lightly, others somewhat darker. The lightly shaded areas need the least amount of work; the darkest areas need the most attention. Work on the lightly shaded areas just once or twice during the course of the treatment; work on the darker areas more frequently, staying at each area no more than 3 to 5 seconds at a time. When you treat an older child, adolescent, or adult, you can locate the acupoints within the darkly shaded areas. But when you treat a baby or young child, working generally in the area of an acupoint will produce the desired result.

Use a gentle touch when you massage your child. When you are working on a baby, all the pressure that's needed is the degree of pressure you would use if you were finger painting or checking to see if a cake is finished baking.

The best time to work on your child is any time he's open to it. Take your time; make him comfortable; relax. This can be fun and pleasurable for both of you. Treatment time combines the joy of connecting with your little one with the pleasure in being able to do something that will help him feel better sooner.

1. Start by gently massaging the chest from the top of the breastbone down toward the stomach.

2. Massage the upper chest, beginning at the center of the upper chest and ending just where the arm meets the chest.

   Massaging the upper chest will help to release the pectoral muscles (pectoralis major and pectoralis minor); these muscles can develop taut bands and trigger points from periods of coughing.

3. Massage in the groove where the chest and the arm meet.

   Lung 1 and Lung 2 are found in the deltopectoral groove, the intersection of the deltoid muscle and pectoralis major. Stimulation of these points will help support lung function.

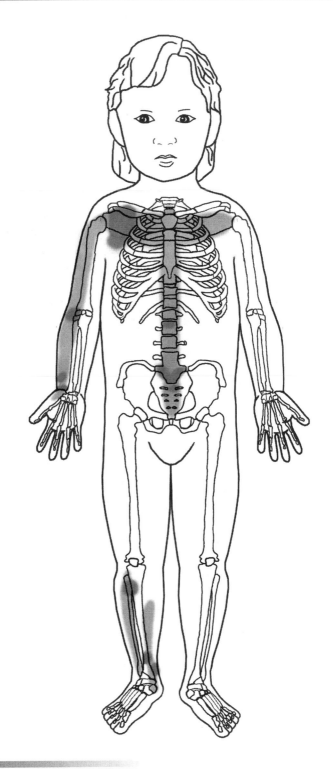

Treatment areas for cold and flu

4. Repeat the massage of the breastbone, this time going all the way down to the lower belly.

5. Apply gentle pressure to the midpoint between the lower end of the breastbone and the belly button.

   Conception Vessel 12 is the point at which the Lung meridian begins.

6. Apply gentle pressure to the point approximately 1 inch below the belly button.

   The combination of the massage of the ribcage and the treatment of Conception Vessel 12 and Conception Vessel 6 helps to open and relax the mid and lower torso, allowing the body to breathe more deeply and easily.

7. Massage the outer part of the front of the arm beginning at the shoulder and working down toward the thumb. Try to focus your massage at the elbow fold, at and just above the wrist, and on the fleshy part of the thumb.

   Lung 5 at the outer part of the elbow fold helps respiration. Lung 7 just above the wrist fold is used to clear congested nasal passages. Lung 9 at the wrist fold and Lung 10 at the center of the thick part of the thumb on the palm side of the hand help support respiratory function.

8. Work on the back side of the hand, between the index finger and the thumb.

   Colon 4 works with Kidney 7 to strengthen immune function.

9. Work on the back of the lower arm just above the wrist fold, in between the two forearm bones.

   Triple Warmer 5 is used in the treatment of the common cold.

10. Massage the outside of the lower leg, giving a bit more attention to the area just beneath the knee.

    Stomach 36 works with Spleen 6 to help strengthen immune function.

11. Work on the inside of the lower leg for several inches above the anklebone.

    Spleen 6 works with Stomach 36 to strengthen the system. Kidney 7 helps support the respiratory process. It works with Colon 4 to strengthen immune function.

12. Massage the upper shoulders an inch or two away from the neck.

    The release of the upper trapezius muscle will help soften the musculature of the neck and shoulders and aid in lymphatic drainage from the neck

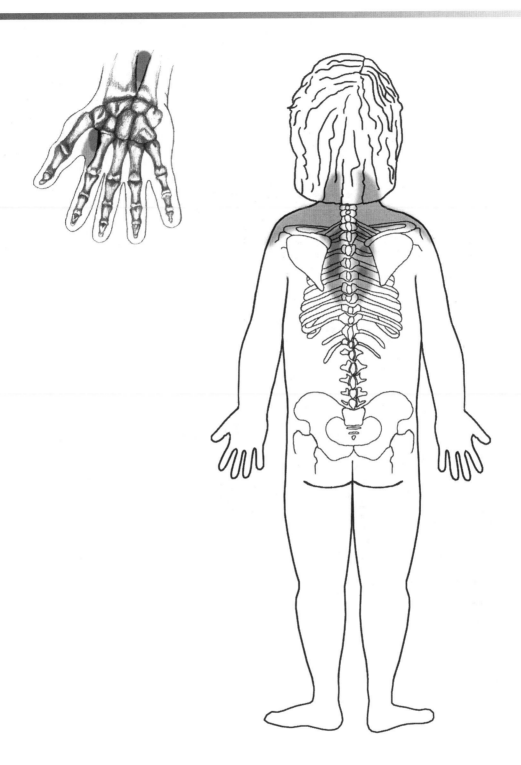

Treatment areas in the upper back and hand for cold and flu

into the upper torso. Each of the yang meridians travels through this area. Their release contributes to the free flow of energy throughout the system.

13. Work on the upper back between the shoulder blades and the spine.

   Bladder 12, 13, and 15 help support the respiratory function. Releasing the muscles of the upper back will help ease breathing.

Working on the face and neck

Massage and acupressure to the face and neck help to open the sinuses and the nasal passages and stimulate lymphatic drainage. The aim is to help your child breathe more easily.

All of these areas should be massaged a couple of times, but do so very, very gently. Your baby or child has a very delicate face, and these points can be quite tender when he's all congested. Light pressure, held for just a couple of seconds, two or three times during the course of a treatment will help him more than you can imagine.

1. Start with a massage of the forehead. Stoke from the bridge of the nose up toward the hairline and then from the midpoint of the forehead out toward the ears.

   Massage of the forehead will help to increase drainage of the frontal and ethmoid sinuses.

2. Gently massage the cheekbones beginning at the nose, just underneath the eyes, and stroke out toward the ears.

   Massage of the cheekbones will help increase drainage of the maxillary sinuses.

3. *Gently* press the point that lies in between the eyebrows.

   Extra point Yintang, at the midpoint of the eyebrows, is commonly used in combination with Taiyang and Colon 4 in the treatment of the common cold.

4. Gently press the area where the eyebrow begins.

   Bladder 2 is used to help clear nasal and sinus congestion.

5. *Gently* press the area midway between the outer edge of the eyebrow and the outer edge of the eye on the temple.

Extra point Taiyang is commonly used in combination with Yintang and Colon 4 in the treatment of the common cold.

6. Gently press beside the nose just above the nostril flare.

   Extra point Bitong is traditionally used to clear nasal congestion.

7. *Gently* press the point just beside each nostril.

   Colon 20 is used to clear congestion in the nasal passages.

8. Massage the neck beginning underneath the ear, stroking downward toward the collarbone.

   A gentle massage of the muscles of the neck, the sternocleidomastoid and the scalenes, will help to increase lymphatic drainage into the upper torso.

9. Massage the top of the collarbone beginning where it meets the breastbone. Massage outwardly toward the shoulder.

   Stomach 11 and 12 are used in the treatment of sore throat. Massage of this area will help to increase lymphatic drainage into the upper torso.

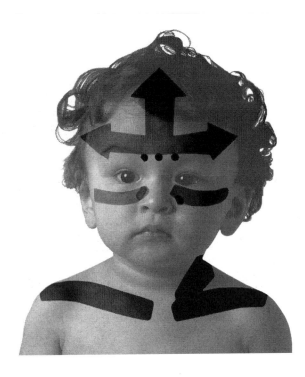

Treatment areas of the face, neck, and temple for the treatment of cold and flu

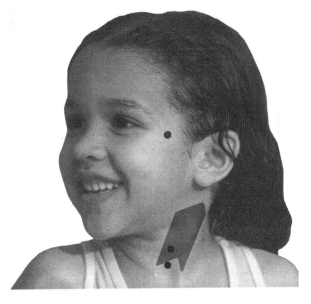

Sore Throat

When should you check with your doctor?

Most sore throats go away by themselves, but you should check with your doctor or health care provider if your child's sore throat is severe and he has a fever of 101.5° F or higher that lasts longer than three or four days. If your baby is drooling excessively it might be a sign of a sore throat that needs to be checked by a doctor. Check with your doctor if your child has difficulty swallowing or breathing or if he has signs of a strep infection: pus (white patches) in the back of his throat or swollen, tender lymph nodes in his neck, a stomach-ache, joint pains, or a rash in addition to a sore throat.

What is it?

We all know what a sore throat is and how it feels. Most adults and children end up with a sore throat at least once or twice a year, usually as part of another illness such as a cold or flu. Sore throats are one of the five most common reasons that children miss school, along with gastroenteritis (stomach flu), colds, conjunctivitis (pink-eye), and ear infections. A sore throat, *pharyngitis,* an inflammation of the pharynx, is frequently the first sign that you're getting sick. We're all familiar with the symptoms—a scratchy or irritated throat that makes swallowing difficult and painful.

What causes it?

Most of the time a sore throat is caused by one of the myriad of viruses that are around during the fall and winter, including the rhinovirus. A sore throat is often the first symptom associated with the onset of a cold or flu. If a virus causes the sore throat, an antibiotic will be of no use. The sore throat will usually go away by itself generally within a week. If the sore throat is the first symptom of a cold, it just might be followed up by the usual: a runny nose, nasal congestion and a cough.

While the vast majority of sore throats are caused by viruses and will resolve themselves, bacteria do cause a small percentage of sore throats. Strep throat, caused by the *Streptococcus* bacteria, is a highly contagious infection of the throat. Like the viruses that cause colds and flu, the strep bacteria are spread through droplets of mucus and saliva sprayed in the air from coughing, sneezing, and speaking or by coming into contact with objects that have been touched by someone who has strep.

Viruses and bacteria are not the only causes of sore throats. Pollutants, secondhand smoke, dust, allergies and dry heat can cause a mild chronically irritated throat.

How do I know if it's strep?

The difference between the way a sore throat feels when it's caused by a virus and when it's caused by strep is often not cut and dry. The information that follows might give you an idea about how strep generally appears, but bear in mind that strep can only be diagnosed by a throat culture that your doctor will do. If you think your child might have a strep infection, take him to the doctor for an exam and a throat culture.

Children between the ages of five and fifteen tend to be more susceptible to strep throats than adults; children younger than three years old rarely get strep. A sore throat caused by strep usually begins with a fever. It's often 101.5° F or higher and it will last several days or until antibiotic treatment has begun. Your child's throat may be red and swollen and his tonsils (the fleshy tissue that lies on the sides of the back of the throat) may be covered with areas of white pus. He will probably have swollen and tender lymph nodes (swollen glands) in his neck. When lymph nodes swell they can feel like firm but spongy beans. You might feel several swollen lymph nodes along the length of his neck. In addition to his throat pain, he may have difficulty swallowing. He may complain of a headache or a stomachache and he won't have an appetite. His joints may ache and he may have a rash. He's likely to seem quite sick—moreso than with a cold.

When your doctor confirms that strep is the cause of your child's sore throat, she will prescribe a course of antibiotics. Once your child starts taking them he'll start to feel better, usually within 24 to 36 hours. If your child is given a course of antibiotics for a strep infection, it's important that he finishes the entire prescription. If strep is not treated with antibiotics it can lead to other infections such as tonsillitis, a sinus infection, or scarlet fever, or serious complications such as inflammation of the kidneys or rheumatic fever, which can damage the heart valves.

How you can help . . .

. . . keep him comfortable

Keep your child home from childcare or school if you think he is contagious, if he still has any fever (even a low-grade fever), or if he is fatigued or "off" and seems to be coming down with something. A day or two at home might prevent your child from getting sicker than he already is and from sharing what he does have with others. If your child is older and has many after-school activities, allow him to skip them while he is recovering.

To ease the pain of a sore throat, teach your child to gargle with salt water.

Gargling with ½ teaspoon of salt in 8 ounces of water will help to ease the throat and clear some mucus.

Sipping warm lemonade or honey and lemon in a cup of warm water helps to ease throat soreness and clear mucus.

Sucking on throat lozenges helps to increase the secretion of saliva, which moistens and eases a sore throat.

Moisten dry air through the use of a humidifier or vaporizer. This will help to soothe a sore, dry, irritated throat. Be sure to clean it regularly and according to manufacturer's directions, in order to maintain its proper functioning.

If your child is particularly uncomfortable or has a fever, speak to your doctor about giving him acetaminophen (Tylenol) or ibuprofen (Advil). Avoid using aspirin with children. It may cause Reye's syndrome, a rare but potentially harmful disease.

In the fall, winter, and early spring, the flu virus is everywhere. So why don't we get colds more often? From the Oriental perspective, if your energy—particularly your *wei chi* (defensive chi)—is strong, your body is easily able to fend off the viruses and bacteria that are all around us all the time. Parents throughout time have warned their children against "getting a draft"—"Put your jacket on, you'll get a cold!" "Keep your head covered." "Don't go out with wet hair—you'll get sick!" Many of us heard these injunctions, or others like them, and probably thought they were nonsense. Well, there's truth in them. Any Oriental medicine practitioner will tell you that the invasion of cold has a negative affect on the body's systems. When it's cold outside, keep your kids warm—keep hats on their heads and socks on their feet, cover their chests, and avoid drafts. Of these, the most important is keeping a hat on their heads—up to 20 percent of your body heat escapes through your head. Something as simple as wearing a baseball cap makes a remarkable difference to total body warmth.

The simplest way to avoid getting sick is to make sure to wash your hands regularly and teach your children to wash theirs. Using soap and warm water or an alcohol-based hand rub (anti-bacterial rubs aren't necessary) is the easiest way to prevent the spread of disease. Colds, the flu, and many other diseases are caused by hand-to-hand contact. Teach your kids to wash after they've touched their face, coughed, or sneezed into their hand or blown their nose if they have a cold. If they don't have a cold, getting one can be prevented if they get into the habit of washing their hands before they eat, after they've used the bathroom, when they come in from playing outdoors, after they've played with or touched the family pet, or after they've been with someone who has a cold. Little things can make the biggest difference.

Teach your children to use tissues to cover their mouth and nose when coughing or sneezing. When tissues are used, make sure to throw them away immediately. If tissues aren't available, teach them to sneeze or cough into the crook of their arm (the bend in their elbow) rather than into their hand. Not only will droplets be prevented from pouring into the air, but there is less of a possibility that they will contaminate objects by touching them with their hands. (If they aren't wearing sleeves, make sure they wash their arms as well as their hands!)

Try to encourage your children to keep their hands, toys, pencils, and anything else that isn't food out of their mouths. Wash toys and other frequently used objects to prevent them from being the source of disease.

Avoid sharing drinking glasses, eating utensils, and towels when someone isn't feeling well. Wash or change drinking glasses (particularly those used in the bathroom) after each use. And be sure to replace his toothbrush after your child has recovered.

A word on diet

When your child has a sore throat, offer him plenty of fluids to keep him well hydrated. Even if he can't swallow large amounts at a time, sipping fluids throughout the day will be soothing to his throat. Chicken broth, herbal teas, diluted juices, and purified water are ideal. Avoid citrus juices, which may irritate an already irritated throat.

Reduce the dairy products you offer your child when he is sick: milk, yogurt, cheeses, ice cream, and puddings. Dairy tends to increase and thicken mucus, which will add to his discomfort. Try substituting soy milk and soy-based cheeses.

Steamed and fresh fruits and vegetables and lightly prepared chicken and fish are easy to digest when your child isn't feeling well.

Avoid high-fat foods such as fried foods, fast foods, or processed or fatty meats, which are difficult to digest (and not very good for him anyway).

As usual, try to keep processed foods and foods that are high in sugars and refined carbohydrates to a minimum.

Treatment

The treatment for a sore throat is aimed at soothing your child's throat, reducing inflammation, and increasing lymphatic drainage. You can use this treatment as soon as your child tells you that his throat hurts. Used once a day during the course of a sore throat or a bout of strep throat, you can help to make your child much more comfortable and increase the speed with which he heals and gets back to being himself.

All of the shaded areas in the treatment illustrations are useful in helping your child to feel better. Some areas are shaded lightly, others somewhat darker. The lightly shaded areas need the least amount of work; the darkest areas need the most attention. Work on the lightly shaded areas just once or twice during the course of the treatment; work on the darker areas more frequently, staying at each area no more than 3 to 5 seconds at a time. When you treat an older child, adolescent, or adult, you can locate the acupoints within the darkly shaded areas. But when you treat a baby or young child, working generally in the area of an acupoint will produce the desired result.

Use a gentle touch when you massage your child. When you are working on a baby, all the pressure that's needed is the degree of pressure you would use if you were finger painting or checking to see if a cake is finished baking.

1. Apply direct gentle pressure to the muscles on the side of your child's neck, starting just behind the sharp angle of the jaw under the ear and moving down toward the collarbone. Work on one side at a time. Press and release in 1/2-inch increments. Hold each point for a count of 2.

   Release of the sternocleidomastoid muscle (SCM) will help to open a sore and tender throat. Gentle downward pressure will help to increase lymphatic drainage of the cervical lymph nodes. Small Intestine 17 and Stomach 9, 10, and 11, lying in front of and along the SCM, are used in the treatment of a sore throat.

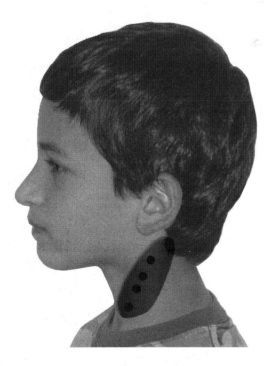

Treatment areas of the neck for sore throat

2. Press gently onto the top of the notch where the collarbones meet, just above the breastbone.

Conception Vessel 22 is used to clear a sore throat.

3. Gently massage along the top of the collarbones. Start at their meeting point in the middle and massage out toward the edge of the shoulder.

Stomach 12, lying at the collarbone behind the SCM, is used to treat a sore throat and to increase lymphatic drainage of the cervical lymph nodes.

4. Gently massage the chest from the top of the breastbone, moving down toward the stomach.

Massage of this area will help bring energy into the torso.

5. Massage the outer edge of the front of the arms from the shoulder down toward the thumb.

Stimulation of the Lung meridian supports respiratory function.

6. Massage the outer edge of the lower arm, just above the wrist.

Lung 7 works with Kidney 6 to reduce inflammation.

7. Massage in the center of the fleshy area of the thumb on the palm side of the hand.

Lung 10 works with Kidney 3 to nourish and strengthen the system.

8. Massage just below the outside edge of the nail on your child's thumb.

Lung 11 is used to clear a sore throat.

9. Massage the back of the hand, between the thumb and the index finger.

Colon 4 is used to clear infection and relieve a sore throat. It works with Kidney 7 to strengthen immune function.

10. Massage the outside of the lower leg, giving a bit more attention to the area just beneath the knee.

Stomach 36 works with Spleen 6 to help strengthen immune function.

11. Work on the inside of the lower leg several inches above the anklebone.

Spleen 6 works with Stomach 36 to strengthen immune function.

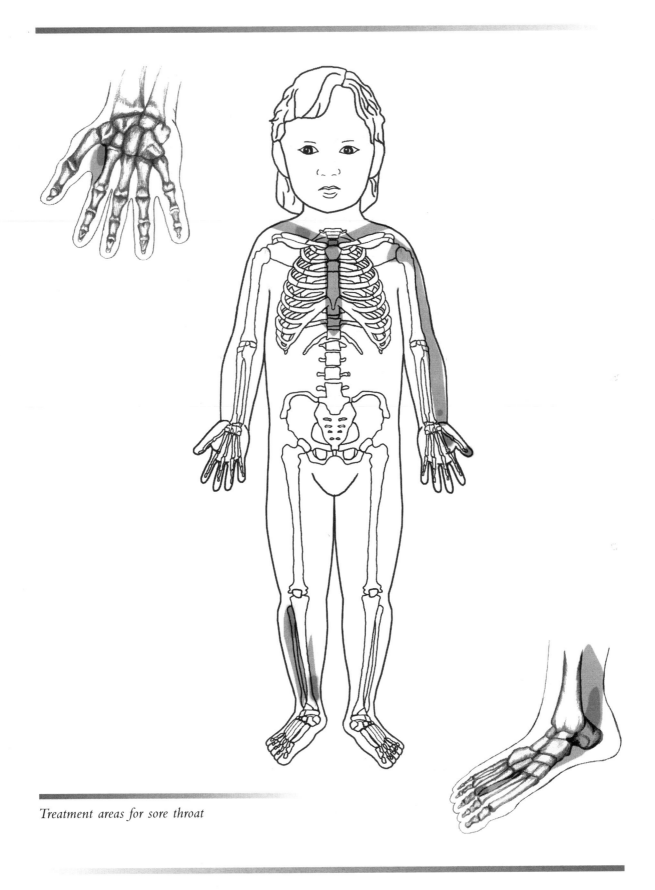

Treatment areas for sore throat

12. Massage around the inside of the anklebone, beginning an inch or so above the bone and working down toward the arch of the foot.

   Kidney 3 is used with Lung 10 to nourish and strengthen the system. Kidney 6 is used with Lung 7 to reduce inflammation. Kidney 7 helps support the respiratory process. It works with Colon 4 to strengthen immune function.

13. Massage in between the long bones leading up to the second and third toes.

   Stomach 43 and 44 are used to clear a sore throat.

14. Massage across the upper shoulders and back.

   Massage of the upper trapezius muscle helps to relieve the neck and upper back stiffness and soreness that may accompany a sore throat. Each of the yang meridians travels through this area. Release of this area contributes to the free flow of energy through the system.

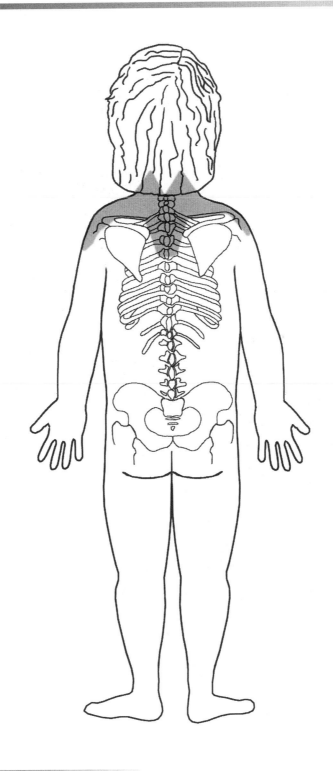

Treatment areas of the back
for sore throat

Ear Infection

When should you check with your doctor?

Consult with your physician if: you suspect that your infant has an ear infection or a fever of 100.4° F; if your child has earache with fever of 102° F or higher, headache, discharge from her ear, swelling around the ear, dizziness, or hearing loss; if your child has had an ear infection that has recurred within two or three weeks; if your child has had more than three ear infections within a six-month period of time.

What is it?

Commonly called an ear infection, *otitis media* is an inflammation of the middle ear. Ear infections are very common in infants and children between the ages of four months and five years. By the age of three, most children will have had at least one ear infection.

Ear infections cause ear pain and fever and can cause temporary hearing loss. If your infant or baby has an ear infection, you may see her pulling on her ear. That's her way of telling you that her ear hurts. She may be irritable and fussy; she may not be able to sleep and she may not want to eat very much. Once she's able to describe how she feels, your child may tell you that her ear hurts or that she feels a fullness or pressure in her ear. Because ear infections may cause temporary hearing loss, you may notice that your child is not hearing sounds as she usually does or is not responding when you speak to her.

What causes it?

An ear infection usually begins with a cold, an upper respiratory infection, or nasal allergies. Colds, sinus problems, and allergies cause swelling and inflammation of the Eustachian tubes, the tubes that connect the middle ear to the back of the nose. Eustachian tubes normally allow fluid to drain out of the middle ear. Eustachian tubes are small, short, and positioned horizontally in children. Swelling and inflammation caused by nasal or sinus congestion will block the tube, trapping fluid inside. Trapped fluid may become a breeding ground for bacteria, leading to an infection. Both the swelling of the Eustachian tube and the pressure caused by the trapped fluid against the eardrum causes pain and, at times, temporary hearing loss.

It's fairly common for fluid to remain within the middle ear for weeks or months after the ear infection is resolved. This is normal and most of the time it clears up on its own. Sometimes, however, this uninfected fluid builds up in the middle ear and remains there. This is called *middle ear effusion*. Middle ear effusion differs from an ear infection in that the child won't have the ear pain and fever associated with an ear infection. If the child has a middle ear effusion the fluid may remain in the middle ear for several months. It's possible that some hearing loss may occur during this time. This is the greatest concern because of the negative impact that hearing loss has on speech development. It is wise to check with your doctor if you suspect that your child's hearing has been impaired.

Will my child need an antibiotic?

Certain ailments require the use of antibiotics: the short list is comprised of strep throat, bacterial pneumonia, some (but not all) ear infections, and sinus infections. Up to this point in time, antibiotics have been used as our first line of defense against disease. The excessive use of antibiotics by humans and the antibiotics that have come into our food supplies through current livestock management has led to more and more powerful bacteria that have grown resistant to the antibiotics we have at hand.

Sometimes when our child is sick, we go to the doctor with the expectation that our child *needs* an antibiotic. Some parents insist on receiving a course of antibiotic therapy for their child. But antibiotics are not needed for every infection. Your doctor is the best judge of that.

Given time, the body can and does heal itself. If we work now to change the way we think about the use of antibiotics, those that we have at our disposal will continue to work against the diseases that we most need them to fight.

How you can help . . .

. . . keep him comfortable

If your child is in pain, applying mild heat to your child's ear may soothe his discomfort. Heat a cup of salt in the oven. Place it in a thin cotton sock. Test it by placing it on the inside of your arm to make sure it is comfortably warm and not too hot. Placing the warmed "salt sock" over your child's ear will help ease the pain of an ear infection. For those of you who tend toward the more modern approaches to life, a beaded microwavable heating pad will do if you make quite sure that it is not too hot when it comes out of the microwave.

Placing 1 or 2 drops of warmed mullein oil in your child's ear will help to reduce swelling and reduce inflammation. If your child won't let you do this while she's awake, place a couple of drops of oil on a small piece of a sterile cotton ball and place it in her ear once she's asleep. If you secure it with a small piece of tape it will work its magic all night.

Rather than prescribing antibiotics, many physicians will take the "watchful waiting" approach to a child's ear infection, knowing that in most cases ear infections will clear up on their own. If your physician believes that this is the best route for your child and yet your child is extremely uncomfortable, you can help alleviate her pain and reduce her fever through the use of over-the-counter pain relievers such as ibuprofen (Advil), acetaminophen (Tylenol), or naproxen sodium (Aleve). Avoid using aspirin. It may cause Reye's syndrome, a rare but potentially harmful disease.

. . . prevent an ear infection

Try to avoid feeding your baby a bottle while she's lying down. Keeping her upright or elevated while she drinks a bottle will help to prevent blocked tubes and the ear infections that might occur as a result.

Keep your children away from secondhand smoke. Children exposed to secondhand smoke tend to experience more ear infections than children who are not.

Think twice about allowing your baby to use a pacifier, particularly between the ages of six and twelve months. Pacifier use has been linked to ear infections in babies in that age group.

A word on diet

Modifying your child's diet will help her to recover quickly. Dairy products tend to thicken and increase the body's mucus production, so avoid giving her any cow's milk or milk products. That includes cheeses, yogurt, cottage cheese, ice cream, and puddings. Try substituting soy milk and soy-based cheeses.

Keep your child well hydrated during the course of her ear infection (and in general). Increasing fluids helps to thin out mucus secretions. Offer her purified water, clear broths, or diluted juices as much as possible throughout the course of the day.

Avoid high fat foods, fried foods, fast foods or fatty or processed meats, which are far more difficult to digest.

And, as always, keep her away from highly processed foods: white sugar (candy, cookies, pastries, sugary drinks), white flour and bread products, and foods laden with chemicals and preservatives.

Treatment

This treatment is aimed at helping you to alleviate your child's discomfort and increase the ability of her body to heal itself. It's likely that if your child has an ear infection she also has some nasal congestion. If this is the case, use the treatment for the common cold (page XX [X-Ref]) in addition to the ear points listed on these pages.

Massage and acupressure to the face and areas surrounding the ear help to open the sinuses, the nasal passages, and the Eustachian tubes. The aim is to help relieve inflammation and increase drainage of the ears. All of these areas should be massaged extremely gently a couple of times. Your child has a delicate face, and these points can be quite tender when she's sick. Very light pressure, held for just a couple of seconds 2 or 3 times during the course of a treatment, will help her more than you can imagine.

All of the shaded areas in the treatment illustrations are useful in helping your child to feel better. Some areas are shaded lightly, others somewhat darker. The lightly shaded areas need the least amount of work; the darkest areas need the most attention. Work on the lightly shaded areas just once or twice during the course of the treatment; work on the darker areas more frequently, staying at each area no more than 3 to 5 seconds at a time. When you treat an older child, adolescent, or adult, you can locate the acupoints within the darkly shaded areas. But when you treat a baby or young child, working generally in the area of an acupoint will produce the desired result.

Use a gentle touch when you massage your child. When you are working on a baby, all the pressure that's needed is the degree of pressure you would use if you were finger painting or using an internal mouse pad on a laptop computer.

Work on your child any time she's relaxed and is ready for a little personal time. Take your time; make her comfortable; relax.

This can be a pleasurable time for both of you. Look at your child when you work on her; smile, talk, play. Treatment time combines the joy of connecting with your little one with the pleasure of being able to do something that will help her feel better sooner.

1. Start with a massage of the forehead. Stoke up from the bridge of the nose toward the hairline and then from midpoint of the forehead out toward the ears.

2. Massage the cheekbones starting at the side of the nose and working out toward the ears.

    Massage of the forehead and face will help to open the sinuses.

3. Massage around the ears, starting at the temple. Work in an arc around the ear and down toward the neck. Use your fingertips to make tiny little circles as you massage this area.

4. Massage from the neck beginning just underneath the ear and gently stroke downward toward the collarbone.

    A gentle massage of the muscles of the neck—the sternocleidomastoid and the scalenes—will help to increase lymphatic drainage into the upper torso.

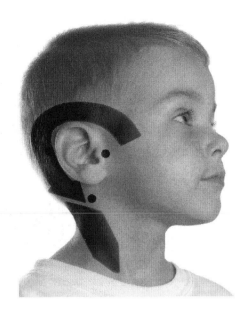

*Treatment areas of the neck
and head for ear discomfort*

5. Place the pad of one finger on the side of the face just in front
    of the "flap" of the ear (the tragus). Hold that point gently for
    a slow count of 5 to 8. (You'll know you're in the right place
    if you feel the top of your child's jaw bone moving under your
    finger when she opens and closes her mouth.)

    *Your finger will encompass three points here: Triple Warmer 21, Small
    Intestine 19, and Gall Bladder 2, all of which help to clear inflamma-
    tion and reduce swelling in the ear.*

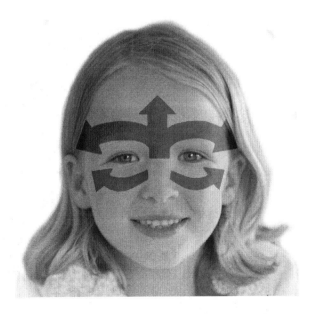

*Treatment areas of the face
and neck for ear discomfort*

6. Gently press the point just behind the ear on the same horizontal line with the tragus of the ear.

   Gall Bladder 11 helps to clear ear inflammation.

7. Gently press the point between the angle of the jaw and the back of the skull just underneath the ear.

   Triple Warmer 17 helps to alleviate ear inflammation.

8. Gently massage the chest. Start at the upper part of the breastbone and massage down toward the stomach. Starting again at the upper part of the breastbone, massage the upper chest out toward the area where the arms meet the upper body. Your fingers will fall into a little space at that area. Give that place a bit of extra attention.

   Lung 1 and Lung 2 are found just in the space where the arm meets the body: the deltopectoral groove, the intersection of the deltoid muscle and pectoralis major. Stimulation of these points will help the respiratory process.

9. Apply gentle pressure to the midpoint between the break in the ribcage and the belly button.

   Conception Vessel 12 is the point at which the Lung meridian begins.

10. Apply gentle pressure to the point approximately an inch below the belly button.

    The combination of the massage of the ribcage and the treatment of Conception Vessel 12 and Conception Vessel 6 helps to open and relax the mid and lower torso, allowing the body to breathe more deeply and easily.

11. Massage the outer part of the front of the arm, from the shoulder down to the thumb. Try to focus your massage on the inside of the arm and the palm of the hand. On the way down pay a bit more attention to the outer part of the elbow fold and the thick part of the thumb on the palm side the hand.

    Lung 5 and Lung 10 support lung function.

12. Massage the back side of his hand between the index finger and the thumb, keeping your pressure slightly closer to the index finger side of the hand.

    Colon 4 helps to support immune function.

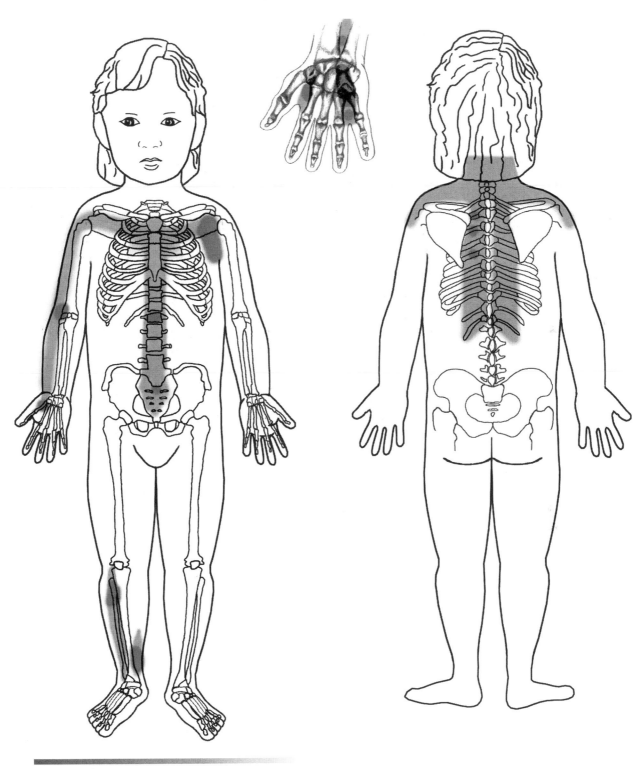

Treatment areas of the front, back,
and hand for ear discomfort

13. Work on the back of the wrist 1 inch or so above the wrist fold, in between the two bones of the forearm just in line with the middle finger.

    Triple Warmer 5 is commonly used in the treatment of ear diseases.

14. Massage the back of the hand between the metacarpals, the long bones connecting to the pinky and ring fingers.

    Triple Warmer 3 is commonly used in the treatment of ear diseases.

15. Massage the outside of the lower leg, giving a bit more attention to the area just beneath the knee.

    Stomach 36 works with Spleen 6 to help strengthen immune function.

16. Work on the inside of the lower leg for several inches above the anklebone.

    Spleen 6 works with Stomach 36 to help strengthen immune function.

17. Massage the top of the shoulders 1 to 2 inches from the neck.

    The release of the upper trapezius muscle will help soften the musculature of the neck and shoulders and aid in lymphatic drainage from the neck into the upper torso. Each of the yang meridians travels through this area. Release of this area contributes to the free flow of energy through the system.

18 Work on the upper back between the shoulder blades and the spine.

    Bladder 12, Bladder 13, and Bladder 15 help respiratory function.

Sinus Infection

When should you check with your doctor?

If your child develops a fever several days into a cold, or if her cold seems to be getting worse rather than better after ten days, your doctor may want to check to see whether a sinus infection has developed. If your child's allergy symptoms are not responding to the allergy medication she's taking, consult with your doctor.

What is it?

A sinus infection, or *sinusitis*, is an infection of the air-filled pockets, or sinuses, that are in the face. Adults have four paired sinuses (each side of the face houses one of each of the four sinuses). Two sinuses are present at birth: the *ethmoid* sinuses at the bridge of the nose and the *maxillary* sinuses above the cheeks. The *frontal* sinuses in the forehead develop at around the age of seven, and the *sphenoid* sinuses, deep in the face, develop during the teen years.

Sound resonates through the sinuses when we speak; air is warmed and moistened in the sinuses when we breathe. Like the nasal passages, the sinus cavities produce and are lined with mucus. Mucus drains through the sinuses into the nasal passages.

Symptoms of a sinus infection are very similar to the symptoms of a cold. But a cold usually improves within a week or so. If your child had a cold and then develops a sinus infection, instead of feeling better after 7 to 10 days of the cold's onset, she'll start to feel worse. She may develop a fever. She might have a runny nose or feel all stuffed up. Her nasal mucus will be a thick green or yellow color, she may have bad breath, swelling around her eyes, and a dry cough caused by a post-nasal drip (mucus running down the back of her throat). The cough might be worse at night, disturbing her sleep. Headaches and facial pain may be present with older kids. Children under seven years old don't generally experience headache because their frontal sinuses are not yet developed.

What causes it?

An inflammation of the mucous membranes due to a cold or allergies can cause a sinus infection. The mucous membranes lining the sinuses swell, blocking the passage of mucus into the nasal passages. Those blocked cavities become a perfect breeding ground for bacteria and viruses.

How you can help . . .

. . . keep her comfortable

If your child is unable to sleep because of a stuffed-up head or a cough due to a post-nasal drip, place a humidifier or vaporizer in her room to help keep her mucous membranes from drying out. Dry air in heated homes during winter months dries out the airways and leads to thicker, stickier mucus. The vaporizer or humidifier will moisten the air, soothe dry mucous membranes, thin out thickened mucus, and make breathing easier. If you do use a humidifier or vaporizer, make sure you clean it regularly according to manufacturer directions.

Place a couple of drops of eucalyptus oil near her pillow to help open a stuffy nose and make breathing easier.

Difficulty sleeping can be due to a cough caused by a *post-nasal drip,* mucus running down the back of her throat. Raise her upper body to help her. If you prop up her upper back and head onto two pillows she'll be able to swallow the mucus more comfortably.

Teach her to breathe deeply and to gently blow her nose while in a steamy bathroom or shower.

If she's particularly uncomfortable or has a fever, speak to your doctor about giving her acetaminophen (Tylenol) or ibuprofen (Advil). Avoid using aspirin with children. It may cause Reye's syndrome, a rare but potentially harmful disease.

. . . prevent a sinus infection

If your child has a cold or an allergy, do all you can do to keep her mucus moving. Nasal saline drops or sprays specially formulated for children help to moisten and clear the nasal passages.

The use of a humidifier or vaporizer in your home helps to moisten the dryness of heated air in the wintertime. Dry heat can dry out and irritate mucous membranes, making them more prone to inflammation. If you do use a humidifier or vaporizer, make sure you clean it regularly according to manufacturer directions.

If your child has had a tendency toward sinus infections, or is she has allergies, keep her in a smoke-free environment.

A word on diet

Dairy products tend to increase the body's production of mucus, so avoid giving her any cow's milk or milk products. That includes cheeses, yogurt, cottage cheese, ice cream, and puddings. Try substituting soy milk and soy-based cheeses.

Increasing fluids helps thin mucous secretions—water, diluted juices, clear broths, and diluted herb teas are all good choices. Try to get her to drink at least 4 ounces every hour.

Steamed and fresh fruits and vegetables and lightly prepared chicken and fish are easy to digest when your child isn't feeling well.

Avoid high fat foods such as fried foods, fast foods, and processed or fatty meats. They tend to be difficult to digest. And, as always, keep her away from highly processed foods: white sugar (candy, cookies, pastries, sodas), white flour and bread products, and foods with chemicals and preservatives.

Treatment

The treatment of your child's head and face will help to open her nasal passages and sinuses and increase lymphatic drainage. The aim is to help her breathe more easily and to reduce inflammation.

All of the areas in the treatment illustrations should be massaged very gently a couple of times. Your child has a delicate face, and these points can be quite tender when she's congested. Extremely light pressure held for just a couple of seconds 2 or 3 times during the course of a treatment will help her more than you can imagine.

If your child has a fever along with her sinus infection, use the treatment for fever on page XX **[X-Ref]** in addition to this treatment, for added benefit.

1. Start with a massage of the forehead. Stoke from the bridge of the nose up toward the hairline and then from the midpoint of the forehead out toward the ears.

    Massage of the forehead will help to increase drainage of the frontal and ethmoid sinuses.

2. Gently massage the cheekbones beginning at the nose, just underneath the eye. Stroke out toward the ears.

    Massaging the cheekbones will help increase drainage of the maxillary sinuses.

3. *Gently* press the area that lies just between the eyebrows.

    Extra point Yintang is commonly used in combination with Taiyang and Colon 4 in the treatment of sinus congestion

4. Gently press the area where the eyebrow begins.

    Bladder 2 is used to help clear nasal and sinus congestion.

5. Gently press the point that lies on the temple midway between the outer edge of the eyebrow and the outer edge of the eye.

    Extra point Taiyang is commonly used in combination with Yintang and Colon 4 in the treatment of sinus congestion.

6. Gently press beside the nose above the nostril flare.

    Extra point Bitong is traditionally used to clear nasal congestion.

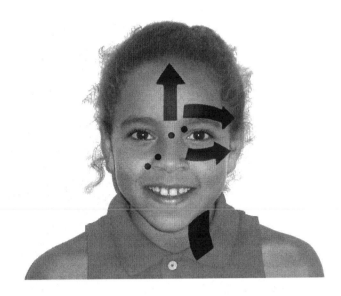

Treatment areas of the face and neck for sinus infection

7. *Gently* press the point just beside each nostril.

   Colon 20 is used to clear congestion in the nasal passages.

8. Massage from the neck beginning underneath the ear and stroke downward toward the collarbone.

   A gentle massage of the muscles of the neck—the sternocleidomastoid and the scalenes—will help to increase lymphatic drainage into the upper torso.

Treatment areas of the temple and neck for sinus infection

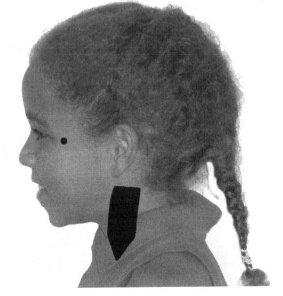

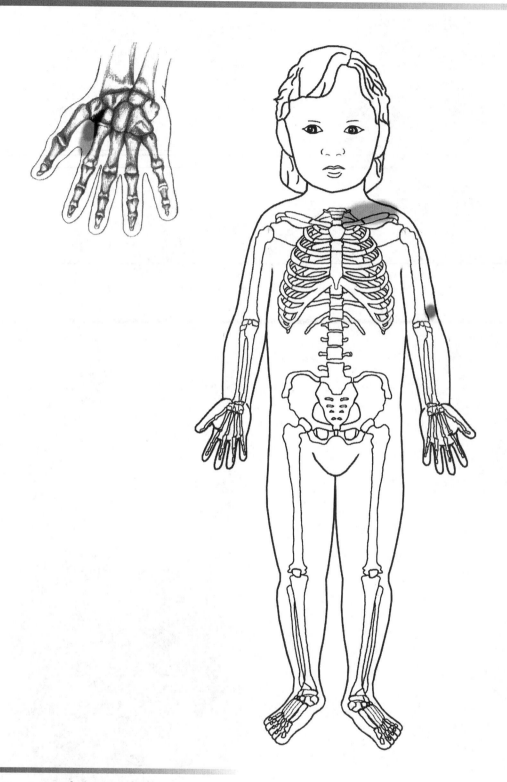

Treatment areas for sinus infection

9. Massage the top of the collarbone, beginning where it meets the breastbone and massaging outward toward the shoulder.

   Massage of this area will help to increase lymphatic drainage into the torso.

10. Massage the point that lies on the outside of the elbow at the place where the elbow creases when you bend the arm.

    Colon 11 is used to treat inflammation and fever.

11. Gently massage the back side of the hand between the index finger and the thumb, Colon 4.

    Colon 4 is commonly used in combination with Yintang and Taiyang in the treatment of sinus congestion.

12. Repeat steps 1 and 2, the gentle stroking of the forehead and cheeks, for a soothing end to the treatment.

Cough

When should you check with your doctor?

See your doctor immediately if your child is coughing up blood, having difficulty breathing, is breathing more rapidly than usual, or if his lips take on a dusky or bluish color. Check with your doctor if your child has a persistent cough that is accompanied by a fever of 102° F or if he has chest pain or is wheezing or making unusual sounds when he breathes. If your baby three months of age or younger has been coughing for more than a few hours, he should be seen by a doctor.

What is it?

A cough is the body's way of clearing its airways—the throat and lungs. Coughing is a reflex, a protective mechanism that moves mucus and other fluids and helps keep the lungs clear of infections. While a cough can sound scary, it's important to remember that most of the time this reflex action is doing what it should to protect the body.

What causes it?

There are many causes of a cough. The most frequent is the common cold or other viral infection, such as the flu. If your child's cough is due to a viral infection, it will go away on its own; antibiotics don't speed the healing of a viral infection. A cough often accompanies a cold, along with nasal congestion and a runny nose. Mucus runs down the back of the throat, producing an irritating and sometimes annoying post-nasal drip. It's this drip that causes the cough. The cough will sound wet and loose, and if the child is old enough he will be able to bring up mucus. If not, he'll swallow quite a bit of mucus. If he does, he may end up vomiting after a coughing spell. Unless the vomiting is persistent, it isn't something you should be concerned about.

Most of the time a cough that is due to a common cold will ease off after four or five days, although it may linger for as long as ten days. If your child seems well and has no fever, he's probably fine, and the cough will go away by itself. But if your little one has developed a fever of 102° F or higher along with his cough and it has lasted more than a three or four days, he should be checked by your doctor just to make sure that the cause of the cough isn't a bacterial infection, such as sinusitis or pneumonia.

Croup causes a cough that sounds like a bark. Both allergies and a viral infection, like a cold or flu, can lead to croup. Croup is an inflammation of the upper airway. The upper airway is the part of the windpipe that is in the throat, the *trachea.* The voice box (the *larynx*) and the airways that lead to the lungs (the *bronchi*) may also be affected by croup. Croup often comes on in the middle of the night, suddenly, when your child is resting or asleep. He may have trouble breathing and his breathing may sound harsh, high-pitched, and noisy. That's called *stridor.* He may have a low-grade fever and his chest might hurt.

Croup generally sounds worse than it is, and because it's a viral infection antibiotics will not help. If your child awakens with a croupy cough, you can help ease his breathing by placing him in a steamy bathroom or near an opened window where he can breathe cool air. Sitting with him in either place will make him a bit more comfortable and get him through the night. If you suspect that your child has croup, check in with your doctor.

Bronchitis is an inflammation of the *bronchi,* the airways in the upper chest that lead to the lungs. Bronchitis in children is most often caused by a viral infection. It may follow a common cold and be referred to as a "chest cold." The dry hacking cough that's typical of bronchitis may last between seven and fourteen days, or possibly longer. Your child may experience a mild fever and some upper chest or back pain along with the cough. As the body starts to heal, the dry cough will become a wetter cough and he'll be able to bring up mucus. That's a good sign—the process is almost over. If you believe your child has bronchitis, check in with your doctor. If his bronchitis is caused by a viral infection, an antibiotic will not help speed the healing process.

Whooping cough, *pertussis,* is a highly contagious bacterial infection. A child who has whooping cough will have severe coughing spells that end with a whooping sound when he breathes in (hence the name). Fortunately, because of the routine use of the DTaP vaccine used to prevent diptheria, tetanus, and acellular pertussis, whooping cough has become far less common than in years past. If your child's cough ends with a whooping sound, or if he's recently been in contact with someone who may have whooping cough, check with your doctor right away. Your doctor will most likely prescribe antibiotics for this bacterial infection.

What is RSV?

Respiratory syncytial virus (RSV) is one of the most common causes of lower respiratory illness in infants and children. It is a highly contagious virus. RSV is usually most active in the winter and early spring months, and is spread, like the flu, through contact with an infected person or something that an infected person has come into contact with. Most kids have been exposed to RSV by the time they are two years old. RSV infections may be quite mild and symptoms will disappear on their own within a few days. However with some children, particularly infants and very young children, RSV can lead to an infection deep in the lungs such as *pneumonia* or *bronchiolitis,* an inflammation of the smallest airways in the lungs.

RSV usually begins with symptoms that are just like those of a cold: stuffy nose, sore throat, and cough. Most generally healthy kids fight it off and it ends there. However, if your child develops bronchiolitis he will have a deep cough and you may be able to hear a wheeze when he breathes out. He may be breathing very rapidly or with difficulty. He may be unwilling to eat and seem very irritable.

If RSV leads to pneumonia, your child may be breathing very fast; he might complain of chest pain along with his cough and he may have a fever.

If you suspect that your child has bronchiolitis or pneumonia, contact your doctor for medical treatment.

How you can help . . .

. . . keep him comfortable

Encourage your child to drink more fluids than he would ordinarily. Fluids will help to thin the mucus, making it easier for him to swallow it or cough it up. Warm fluids are ideal—try warm lemonade or mild ginger or herbal tea sipped throughout the day. Avoid giving him acidy juices such as orange juice, which can irritate a throat that is already irritated from coughing.

Keep your child home from childcare or school if you think he is in a contagious phase of a cold, of he has any fever at all (even a low grade fever) or if he is fatigued or "off" and seems to be coming down with something. A day or two at home might prevent your child from getting sicker and from sharing his cold with others. If your child is older and has many after-school activities, allow him to skip them while he is recovering from a cold as well.

If you are allowing the child to stay home from school, keep him in an area where the temperature is warm and stable. And let him rest. Rest and sleep are the greatest healers. The body knows it.

If your child is having difficulty breathing at night or he's unable to sleep because of a cough, use a vaporizer or humidifier to moisten the air. Dry air in heated homes during winter months dries out the airways and leads to thicker, stickier mucus. The vaporizer or humidifier will moisten the air, soothe dry mucous membranes, thin out thickened mucus, and make breathing easier. If you do use a humidifier or vaporizer, make sure you clean it regularly according to manufacturer directions.

If your child wakes up with a croupy cough, sit with him in a steamy bathroom for 15 or 20 minutes. The moistness of the air will help him breathe more easily. Placing him near an opened window where he can breathe cool, fresh air can also help to ease his coughing.

Antibiotics will not speed the healing of a viral infection. Questions abound about the value of antihistamines, decongestants, cough suppressants, and many other over-the-counter preparations. If your child's cough is due to a cold or virus, let it run its course unless your doctor suggests that you do otherwise. If your child is uncomfortable or has a fever, speak to your doctor about giving him acetaminophen (Tylenol) or ibuprofen (Advil). Avoid using aspirin with children. It may cause Reye's syndrome, a rare but potentially harmful disease.

... prevent him from getting sick

The best way to prevent the spread of disease is to wash your hands regularly and to teach your children to wash theirs well and often. Using soap and warm water or an alcohol-based hand rub is the easiest way to prevent the spread of disease. (Anti-bacterial soaps or hand rubs aren't necessary and may in fact promote the growth of antibiotic-resistant bacteria.) Colds, the flu, and many other viruses and diseases are caused by hand-to-hand contact. Teach your kids to wash after they've touched their face, coughed or sneezed into their hand, or blown their nose if they have a cold. Getting sick can be prevented if our kids get into the habit of washing their hands before they eat, after they've used the bathroom, when they come in from playing outdoors, after they've played with or touched the family pet, or after they've been with someone who has a cold. Little things can make the biggest difference.

Teach your children to use tissues to cover their mouth and nose when coughing or sneezing. When tissues are used, make sure to throw them away immediately. If tissues aren't available, teach them to sneeze or cough into the crook of their arm (the bend in their elbow) rather than into their hand. Not only will droplets be prevented from pouring into the air, but there is less of a possibility that your children will contaminate objects by touching them with their hands. (If they're not wearing sleeves, make sure they wash their arms also!)

Try to encourage your children to keep their hands, toys, pencils, and anything else that isn't food out of their mouths.

Wash toys and other objects frequently, including remote controls, computer keyboards, and telephones, to prevent them from being the source of disease. Avoid sharing drinking glasses, eating utensils, and towels when someone in your household has a cold. Wash or change drinking glasses, including those used in the bathroom, after each use. Replace your child's toothbrush after he has recovered.

A word on diet

Modifying your child's diet will help him recover quickly. Dairy products tend to increase the body's mucus production, so avoid giving him any cow's milk or milk products. That includes cheeses, yogurt, cottage cheese, ice cream, and puddings. Try substituting soy milk and soy-based cheeses.

Increasing fluids helps thin mucous secretions—give your child water, diluted juices, clear broths, and diluted herb teas to drink. Chicken soup really does do wonders!

Steamed and fresh fruits and vegetables and lightly prepared chicken and fish are easy to digest when your child is sick.

Avoid high fat foods, fried foods, and fatty or processed meats, which are difficult to digest, particularly if your child tends to vomit after a coughing spell. And, as always, keep him away from highly processed foods: white sugar (candy, cookies, pastries, sugary drinks), white flour and bread products, and foods laden with chemicals and preservatives.

Treatment

Regardless of the type of cough your child has, a treatment will help to relax the muscles of his chest and ease his breathing. If your child's cough seems to be coming from nasal congestion or a post-nasal drip, use the sinus treatment on page XX in addition to this one.

All of the shaded areas in the treatment illustrations are useful in helping your child to feel better. Some areas are shaded lightly, others somewhat darker. The lightly shaded areas need the least amount of work; the darkest areas need the most attention. Work on the lightly shaded areas just once or twice during the course of the treatment; work on the darker areas more frequently, staying at each area no more than 3 to 5 seconds at a time. When you treat an older child, adolescent, or adult, you can locate the acupoints within the darkly shaded areas. But when you treat a baby or young child, working generally in the area of an acupoint will produce the desired result.

Use a gentle touch when you massage your child. When you are working on a baby, all the pressure that's needed is the degree of pressure you would use if you were finger painting or checking to see if a cake is finished baking. The best time to work on your child is any time he's open to it. Take your time; make him comfortable; relax. This can be fun and pleasurable for both of you.

1. Begin with a gentle massage of the chest. Start at the upper part of the breastbone and massage down toward the upper stomach.

2. Starting again at the upper part of the breastbone, massage the upper chest out toward the area where the arms meet the upper body. Your fingers will fall into a little space just at that place. Give that place just a little extra attention.

   When you cough, the chest muscles will naturally get somewhat constricted. Massaging these areas will help to release the pectoral muscles (pectoralis major and pectoralis minor) which can develop taut bands and trigger points from extended periods of coughing. Lung 1 and Lung 2 are found in the deltopectoral groove, the intersection of the deltoid muscle and pectoralis major where the arm meets the body. Stimulation of these points will help the respiratory process.

3. Apply very gentle pressure to the points that lie in between the rib spaces, where the ribs meet the breastbone.

   Kidney 22—Kidney 26 are commonly used to treat cough and other respiratory conditions.

4. Massage the lower part of the ribcage from the center out toward the sides of the body.

   The abdominal and pectoral muscles interconnect at this area. Release of the tissues in this area will help your child to breathe deeply.

5. Apply gentle pressure to the midpoint between the break in the ribcage and the belly button.

   Conception Vessel 12 is the point at which the Lung meridian begins.

6. Apply gentle pressure to the point approximately 1 inch below the belly button.

   Conception Vessel 6 opens the "sea of energy" in the lower warmer. The combination of the massage of the ribcage and the treatment of Conception Vessel 12 and Conception Vessel 6 helps to open and relax the mid and lower torso, allowing the body to breathe more deeply and easily.

7. Massage the outside of the front of the arms. Apply gentle pressure at the area of the elbow fold; at the lower part of the bulge of the forearm, about 1/3 of the way down the arm; at 1 inch or so above the wrist; and at the wrist fold.

   Lung 5 is used to relieve cough and increase deep breathing. Lung 6 is used at the onset of respiratory ailments. Lung 7 is commonly used along with Conception Vessel 22 in the treatment of cough. Lung 9 is commonly used along with Colon 4 in the treatment of respiratory problems.

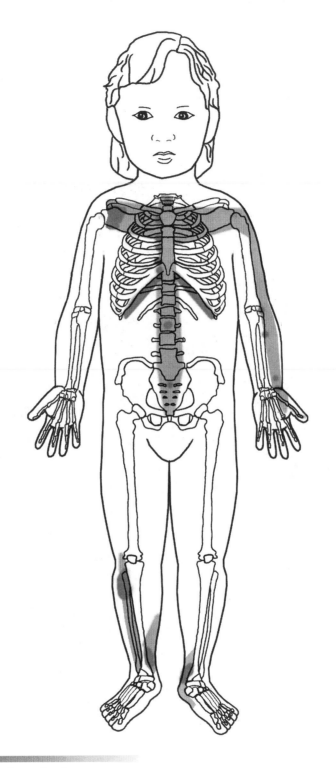

Treatment areas for cough on the front

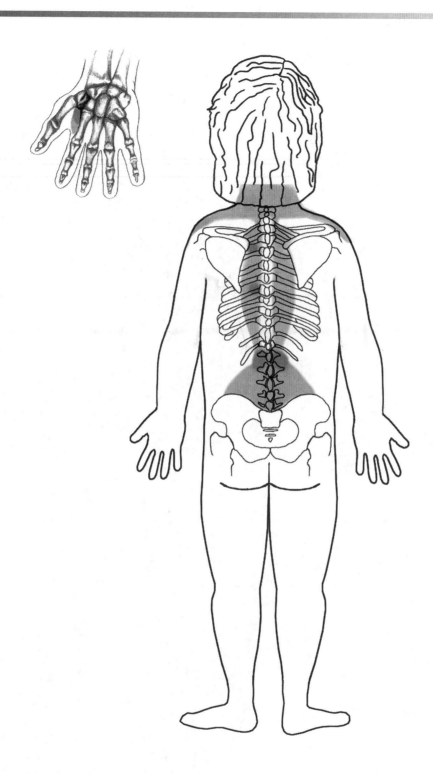

Treatment areas for cough on the back and hand

8. Gently massage the back side of the hand between the index finger and the thumb.

   Colon 4 is commonly used with Lung 9 in the treatment of respiratory problems. Colon 4 works with Kidney 7 to strengthen immune function.

9. Apply very gentle pressure onto the top of the notch where the collarbones meet, just above the breastbone.

   Conception Vessel 22 is commonly used along with Lung 7 in the treatment of cough.

10. Massage the outside of the lower leg, giving a bit more attention to the area just beneath the knee.

    Stomach 36 works with Spleen 6 to help strengthen immune function.

11. Work on the inside of the lower leg, several inches above the anklebone.

    Spleen 6 works with Stomach 36 to strengthen immune function.

12. Massage around the inside of the anklebone, beginning 1 inch or so above it and working down toward the arch of the foot.

    Kidney 7 helps support the respiratory process. It works with Colon 4 to strengthen immune function.

13. Massage the top of the shoulders, 1 or 2 inches from the neck.

    The release of the upper trapezius muscle will help soften the musculature of the neck and shoulders and aid in lymphatic drainage from the neck into the upper torso. Each of the yang meridians travels through this area. Releasing this area contributes to the free flow of energy through the system.

14. Gently massage the area between the shoulder blades and the spine, focusing on the areas just beside the upper part of the shoulder blade and its lowest part.

    Bladder 13, beside the spine of the scapula, and Bladder 17, beside the inferior angle of the scapula, are commonly used in the treatment of cough.

15. Gently massage the lower back from the bottom of the ribcage to the upper part of the pelvis.

    Quadratus lumborum, deep in the lower back, often becomes restricted due to coughing. Release of the muscle will help to ease breathing. Bladder 23 and Bladder 52 will help to strengthen the system.

Asthma

When should you check with your doctor?

An acute asthma attack can be medical emergency! Call 911 or take your child to the emergency room if his wheezing or coughing is severe and he is unable to catch his breath, if he is breathing very rapidly or so hard that he is using his abdominal muscles to breathe, if his nostrils flare out when he breathes, if he is having difficulty speaking because of shortness of breath, if he complains of chest tightness or pain, or if his lips or fingernails are turning blue.

Your child should be evaluated by your physician if he is having difficulty breathing due to coughing or wheezing, if he appears to be short of breath, or if he describes a tightness or a "funny feeling" in his chest.

Consult with your doctor if your child's colds always seem to end up as "chest colds"; if exercise, play, laughter and tantrums lead to episodes of coughing or wheezing; or if he frequently awakens in the middle of the night with a dry cough or wheeze.

What is it?

Asthma is the most common chronic, persistent, childhood disease. In the course of the latter part of the twentieth century, it became much more widespread. A cure has yet to be found for asthma, but asthma can almost always be managed and controlled. Working with your physician, you can educate yourself about your child's condition and its specific triggers. You can come to understand how asthma manifests in your child and develop a treatment plan in order to control it. The vast majority of children with asthma can and do lead normal, happy lives.

Asthma, also known as *reactive airway disease*, is a chronic inflammation of the airways of the lungs—the bronchial tubes and smaller bronchioles. Inflammation of the airways causes them to be hyperreactive to the presence of substances in the air, such as allergens, irritants, and pollutants, substances that are around us all the time. Inflamed airways are more prone to react to the presence of irritants with an increased secretion of mucus, swelling of the mucous membranes that line the airways, and contraction of the muscles that form the airways. The end result is a narrowing of the airways, which obstructs the free flow of air. It is this narrowing that makes breathing difficult. Air is blocked from moving freely in and out of the lungs. It is this blockage that produces the characteristic cough or wheeze associated with asthma.

This inflammatory process takes place in everyone who's exposed to irritants to one degree or another. However, when a person has asthma their airways overreact. An asthma attack can lead to significant shortness of breath and low oxygen levels in the blood.

The most common symptoms of asthma are coughing, wheezing (a high-pitched whistling sound that you may or may not be able to hear), difficulty breathing, shortness of breath, and a dry, unproductive cough that keeps the child up at night. More subtle signs of asthma in a child are chest tightness, difficulty sleeping, and not being able to keep up with the other kids at play because of breathing problems.

Asthma is a chronic condition; it has no cure, and the symptoms may persist for months and even years at a time. A child's asthma symptoms may get better at times, but they don't completely go away. A small percentage of children seem to outgrow their asthma as they enter into their adolescent and young adult years. It is unclear which children will fall into this group and which children won't. If you're wondering whether or not your child has asthma, ask yourself these questions about your child's behavior.

- Has your child had frequent or recurrent breathing problems over the past months or year?
- Do you hear your child wheeze when he breathes?

- Does he seem to cough frequently, particularly at night?
- Does exercise, play, or laughing make him cough?
- When he gets a cold does it go right into a cough and does the cough seem to last a very long time, regardless of the medications he is given?
- Does he have frequent or recurrent colds or coughs?
- Has he had pneumonia or bronchiolitis?
- Does he or someone in your family have allergies?
- Does he have eczema?
- Do strong smells such as perfume or tobacco smoke make him cough?
- Does he cough when he gets excited, cries, or has a temper tantrum?
- Does he often complain that his chest hurts or feels funny?
- Do his chest and neck muscles seem unusually tight for a child his age?
- Does he sometimes sound as if he's short of breath?
- Does he seem to breathe very rapidly?

If you've answered yes to several of these questions, discuss your child's symptoms with your doctor. She will be able to diagnose asthma more easily with the older child through the use of pulmonary function tests, tests that measure the lungs' ability to take in air.

What causes it?

Most children who develop asthma tend to be highly allergic and have family members who have allergies and who may have asthma as well. *Allergens* (things that cause allergies), *irritants,* and *weather changes* are common triggers for asthma.

Some very common *indoor allergens*—dust mites, feathers, mold, pet dander, and cockroach debris—can be triggers for someone who has asthma. *Outdoor allergens* that trigger asthma include mold and pollen. The most common *food allergens* are cow's milk, wheat, soy, eggs, peanuts, and tree nuts. Food allergies don't often trigger a full-blown asthma attack. However, they may cause mild allergic reactions, which, over time, cause ongoing low-level inflammation of the airways. This may lead to greater sensitivity and reactivity to other inhaled allergens or irritants. If you believe that your child has allergies that trigger his asthma, speak to your doctor about allergy testing so you can reduce the possible culprits that are making life difficult for your little one.

Irritants, substances that irritate the airways and trigger asthma, include cigarette and cigar smoke, pollutants in the air, and strong smells such as paint fumes and perfumes. While air pollution may not necessarily be avoided, we can limit our exposure to cigarette smoke, paint fumes, perfumes, and other harsh odors.

Weather conditions can trigger asthma: cold air, spring pollen, mold in the fall.

In addition to allergens and irritants, *exercise* often triggers asthma—running around with other kids or playing a group sport can trigger an asthma attack. So does having a cold or other *viral infection* or a chronic sinus infection.

Asthma has many triggers. Some you can help to avoid; some you cannot. Even so, coupling keen observation of your child with a working treatment plan developed with your physician, your child's asthma can be managed well.

How you can help

Watch your child carefully to note the first hints of breathing difficulty. Be a calming force for a child who may fear his asthma and be fearful of having an asthma attack. Know that you can help him; know that as he gets older you can help him learn to help himself. Teach him what he needs to do for himself and work with him to help him understand the importance and value of each of the things that will be helpful to him.

Work with a physician you know and trust to establish an action plan aimed at controlling your child's asthma. The purpose of controlling asthma is not just for reducing daily symptoms, but for reducing the level of airway inflammation that leads to obstruction and an asthma attack as well. An action plan will also give you a clear idea of what to do should your child have an asthma attack.

Have your child tested for allergies to determine which substances are triggers for his asthma. That will help define what he should avoid.

Ban cigarette and cigar smoking around your child and avoid taking him into situations where he may be exposed to secondhand smoke.

If you use a fireplace in your home, have your chimney and flue cleaned regularly to ensure their proper function.

Try to avoid exposing your child to the dust and debris associated with household construction projects, including painting and refinishing floors.

Keep your child away from the fumes from solvents: paints, non-water based glues, furniture strippers, gasoline fumes, perfumes, nail polish, and nail polish remover.

Clean and vacuum your home regularly and carefully to get rid of dust (and therefore dust mites), pet hair, and dander. This includes cleaning carpets, drapes, throw pillows, and stuffed animals.

Use an allergy-proof mattress cover on his mattress and pillows. Wash his bedding regularly.

Keep your child away from mold-producing areas, including basements, damp leaves, and garden debris. Avoid being outdoors when pollen, pollution, or ozone levels are unusually high.

Encourage him to drink fluids throughout the day; water, diluted juices, herbal teas, and broths—fluids will thin any mucous secretions and help him move them out of his bronchial tubes, ultimately helping him to breathe.

Encourage physical activity when your child's asthma is controlled and his symptoms are minimal. His lungs will become conditioned and more efficient through the use they get through physical exercise.

A word on diet

The components of the foods that we ingest make up the components of our bodies. Consider this notion—My body is made up of the same stuff that this earth is made of by some force far greater than me. My body is trying to contend with a chronic disease. How should I best nourish it? How should I take care of it?

In my mind it is essential to give the body the nutrients that needs, avoiding the substances that the body cannot digest and assimilate with ease. I believe that foods that are grown naturally are best for all of us, but are especially so for those who are dealing with a chronic disease.

Please try to feed your child whole foods; foods that are organic are produced without chemical fertilizers, antibiotics, hormones, or growth modifiers; they do not contain GMOs (genetically modified organisms), chemicals, preservatives or additives; they are not distorted or transformed by any means. They are foods as nature intended them to be. Organic foods are more easily obtained these days. To the extent that you can, try to include them in your child's diet, and in your diet.

The most common food allergens are cow's milk (and therefore all the foods that are made from cow's milk), wheat, soy, eggs, peanuts, and tree nuts. Even if your child does not appear to be allergic to any foods, I believe that it would be wise to limit his consumption of these foods. If your child is allergic or sensitive to any particular food, that food should be eliminated from his diet.

The following are suggestions for a healthful diet.

- Feed your kids (and yourself) a well-balanced, varied diet.
- Complete proteins such as lean cuts of beef and pork, poultry, fish, eggs, and low fat dairy products are important for tissue development. Naturally or organically produced meats, poultry, eggs, and dairy are grown both humanely and without the use of antibiotics and hormones. They are a good choice if you can find them. Your child may not be allergic to dairy products; however, many people find that cow's milk and milk products increase their mucus production. Try to limit the dairy products that your child consumes (milk, cheese, yogurt, ice cream, and puddings). You might try replacing them with soy milk or rice milk products.
- Beans, soy, nuts, and whole grains are good vegetable sources of protein and should be part of a healthy diet.
- Choose organically produced fruits and vegetables that are locally grown and in season.
- Eat a diet that includes whole grains and whole grain products: wheat, oats, brown rice, barley, quinoa. Products that are made from organic ingredients and do not contain chemical additives and preservatives are best.
- Limit your child's consumption of refined carbohydrates, white flour, and white sugar products. Some foods really should be special occasional treats: sugared cereals, cookies, pastries, candy, and sugared drinks such as sodas and drink mixes. Many of these foods are high in calories and have little nutrient value.

- Limit your child's consumption of fast foods, fried foods, and junk foods. Between the questionable nutritional quality and the high amounts of salt and saturated fats, you'll be doing your kids a favor if you make these foods very occasional treats.
- Avoid the use of prepackaged, prepared foods and foods that contain preservatives and chemical additives. It's so important to read food labels. If you can't pronounce an ingredient, it's likely that it's an artificial additive.
- Encourage your children to drink purified water and diluted fruit juices. Babies and young children should have no more than 4 to 6 ounces of fruit juice daily. They are often high in sugar. When kids fill up on juices they often don't have room left over for more nutritious foods.

Treatment

This treatment is designed to strengthen your child's immune system. It will help to reduce inflammation, strengthen his breathing, and calm him. The treatment will relax the muscles of his chest, abdomen, neck, and back—it's the muscles in those areas that tighten up so much when he has difficulty breathing. Once they get tight, they don't let go without a bit of intervention.

This treatment is not designed to stop an asthma attack; its aim is to help reduce inflammation and encourage normal breathing. In other words, use it as a means by which you can help your child strengthen his system. It is another tool that you can use to help him control his asthma. Like so many other tools for healthy living, it can be quite a powerful one when used regularly, once or twice weekly, Over time the value of this treatment will become clear when you see that your child needs to use his medications less frequently.

All of the shaded areas in the treatment illustrations are useful in helping your child to feel better. Some areas are shaded lightly, others somewhat darker. The lightly shaded areas need the least amount of work; the darkest areas need the most attention. Work on the lightly shaded areas just once or twice during the course of the treatment; work on the darker areas more frequently, staying at each area no more than 3 to 5 seconds at a time. When you treat an older child, adolescent, or adult, you can locate the acupoints within the darkly shaded areas. But when you treat a baby or young child, working generally in the area of an acupoint will produce the desired result.

Use a gentle touch when you massage your child. When you are working on a baby, all the pressure that's needed is the degree of pressure you would use if you were finger painting or checking to see if a cake is finished baking.

The best time to work on your child is any time he's open to it. Take your time; make him comfortable; relax.

Start your treatment with your child lying on his back. Position yourself behind his head so you can massage his neck easily. Once you've done that you can move so your body is facing his.

1. Massage the neck muscles starting under the ears and working down toward the collarbone.

   The sternocleidomastoid and the scalene muscles elevate the ribcage during breathing. When breathing is labored or difficult, these muscles overwork and may constrict more readily. Massaging this area helps to release these muscles.

2. Massage gently, but deeply, at the base of the skull.

   Gall Bladder 20 is used in the treatment of asthma.

3. Gently massage the muscles of the chest and ribcage. Massage down the center of the chest from the upper part of the breastbone down through his stomach.

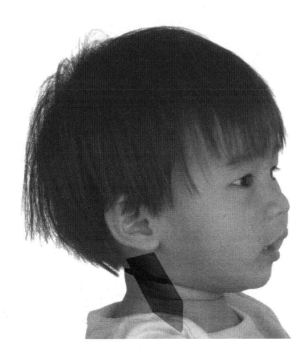

Treatment areas of the neck for asthma

Massage here will bring energy down from the upper chest and into the lower part of the torso.

4. Massage out from the center of the chest to where the arms meet the body.

    Pectoralis major tends toward tightening in response to difficult breathing. Lung 1 and Lung 2 are found in the deltopectoral groove, the space where the arm meets the body at the intersection of the deltoid muscle and pectoralis major. Stimulating these points will help support lung function.

5. Massage the sides of the ribcage, beginning just underneath the arm and working down toward the bottom of the ribcage. Keep your palms flat on the body as you work. It will help prevent you from tickling this very sensitive area.

    Serratus anterior will develop trigger points with excessive coughing. The Gall Bladder channel lies on the side of the upper torso. Manipulation here will tend to be very calming to the system. Spleen 21 is called the universal connecting (luo) point. It will help to balance yin and yang.

6. Massage the edges of the ribcage, starting where the ribs separate from the breastbone and massaging out toward the sides.

    The abdominal and pectoral muscles interconnect at this area. Release of the tissues in this area will help your child to breathe deeply.

7. Apply very gentle pressure onto the top of the notch where the collarbones meet, just above the breastbone.

    Conception Vessel 22 is commonly used along with Lung 7 in the treatment of cough.

8. Apply very gentle pressure to the points that lie in between the rib spaces, where the ribs meet the breastbone.

    Kidney 22–Kidney 26 are commonly used to treat conditions of the lungs.

9. Gently press the breastbone right in between the nipples.

    Conception Vessel 17 helps to open breathing and calm the body.

10. Gently press the point on the midline approximately 1 inch below the place where the ribs separate from the breastbone.

    Conception Vessel 15 helps to relieve the feeling of fullness in the chest.

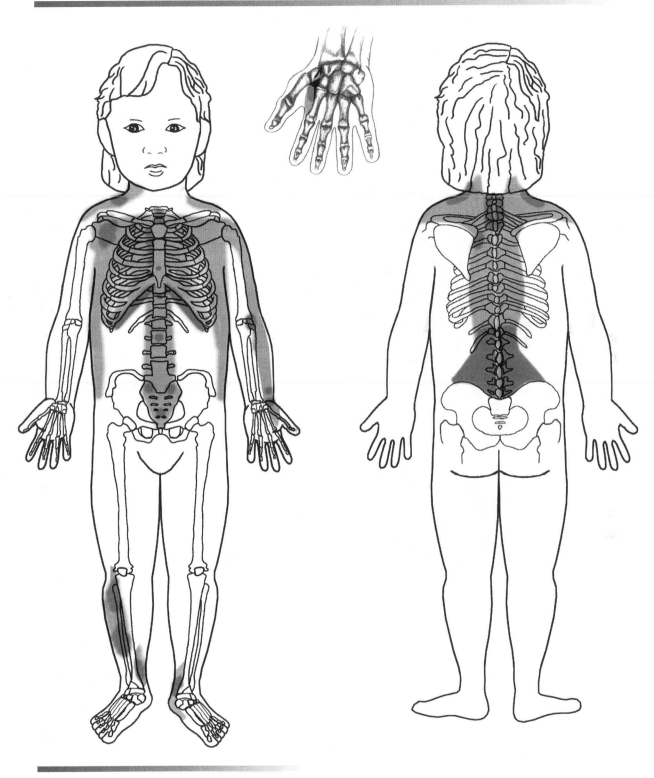

Treatment areas of the front, back, and hand for asthma

11. Gently press the point midway between the belly button and the break in the ribcage right on the midline.

    Conception Vessel 12 helps to strengthen the system.

12. Massage the tops of the shoulders, starting where the neck meets the shoulders and working out to where the shoulders meet the arms.

    Upper trapezius will tend to become constricted during labored breathing. Massage here will help to release upper trapezius. Gall Bladder 21, located at the high point at the top of the shoulder, is used in the treatment of asthma.

13. Massage the outside part of the front of the arm, beginning at the shoulder and working down to the fleshy part of the thumb.

    Following the pathway of the Lung meridian supports lung function.

14. Gently press the point on the outside edge of the elbow fold on the front of the arm.

    Lung 5 is used to restore deep breathing

15. Gently press the point 1 inch or so above the wrist fold on the thumb side of his hand.

    Lung 7 is used to restore deep breathing. It is used with Conception Vessel 22 in the treatment of respiratory problems.

16. Gently press the point on the wrist fold where the thumb meets the hand.

    Lung 9 is used to strengthen the lungs. It is used with Colon 4 in the treatment of respiratory problems.

17. Gently massage the area on the wrist fold where the pinky meets the hand.

    Heart 7 helps calm the mind.

18. Gently massage the back side of the hand between the index finger and the thumb.

    Colon 4 is commonly used with Lung 9 in the treatment of respiratory problems.

19. Massage the lower belly starting just below the belly button.

    Conception Vessel 4 helps to strengthen the system.

20. Gently press the point just beside the belly button.

    Kidney 16 is used to strengthen immune function.

21. Massage the outside of the front of the lower leg from underneath the knee to the ankle. Focus on the area a couple of inches below the knee and in the middle of the lower leg.

    Stomach 36 and Stomach 40 will help strengthen the system. Stomach 36 is used with Spleen 6 to help strengthen immune function.

22. Massage the inside of the lower leg a few inches above the anklebone.

    Spleen 6 is used with Stomach 36 to help strengthen immune function.

23. Massage around the inside of the anklebone, beginning 1 inch or so above the ankle and working down toward the arch of the foot.

    Kidney 7 helps support the respiratory process. It works with Colon 4 to strengthen immune function.

24. Massage the top of the shoulders, focusing in the area 1 to 2 inches from the neck.

    The release of the upper trapezius muscle will help soften the musculature of the neck and shoulders. Each of the yang meridians travels through this area. Its release contributes to the free flow of energy through the system. Gall Bladder 21, at the high point in the muscle at the top of the shoulder, is used in the treatment of asthma. Massage surrounding C7–T1, the area closest to the spine where the neck meets the upper back, is traditionally used in the treatment of asthma.

25. Massage the back beginning at the shoulders and working down both sides of the spine toward the low back and pelvis. Focus on the upper back and the small of the back, the area just above the pelvis.

26. Gently press the point just beside the top of the shoulder blade.

    Bladder 13 beside the spine of the scapula is used in the treatment of respiratory disorders.

27. Gently press the points that lie between the end of the ribcage and the pelvis beside the upper part of the lumbar spine.

    Bladder 23 and Bladder 52, at the level of the second lumbar vertebra, help to strengthen the system. Quadratus lumborum, deep in the lower back, often becomes restricted due to coughing. Release of the muscle will help to ease breathing.

Conjunctivitis

When should you check with your doctor?

Infectious conjunctivitis is highly contagious. If you suspect that your child has conjunctivitis or any eye infection, see your physician to confirm the diagnosis. If your child's eye is irritated, inflamed, red, or swollen for more than twenty-four hours; if your child complains of eye pain, sensitivity to light, or unusual blurred, poor vision; or if he is blinking or tearing excessively, see your doctor.

What is it?

Conjunctivitis, or "pinkeye" as it is commonly called, is an inflammation of the clear, thin membrane that surrounds the eye and lies under the eyelid, the conjunctiva. The term *pinkeye* describes what happens with conjunctivitis—the white part of the eyeball will appear pink or red. Your child might tell you that she feels as though she has something in her eye, and her eye might tear quite a lot. When she wakes up in the morning her eye might feel as though it is "glued shut," and indeed it might be crusted over and difficult to open, due to the discharge that comes from the eye as a result of the inflammation. She might experience soreness or itchiness in her eye and may possibly experience blurred vision, along with some sensitivity to light.

Conjunctivitis is fairly common in children. It is one of the five most common reasons—along with sore throat, colds, ear infections and stomach flu— that children miss school. Conjunctivitis can affect one or both eyes and it can be highly contagious. A child can be contagious for up to two weeks after their symptoms first appear.

What causes it?

Conjunctivitis is most commonly caused by a virus, but it can also be caused by bacteria or an allergy. Both the viral and the bacterial forms of conjunctivitis are highly contagious and are spread through direct contact with someone who has it. Unfortunately, conjunctivitis is quite common in children and, because they are children, it is quite easily spread amongst them.

Viral conjunctivitis causes a watery or mucous discharge from the eye. Viral pinkeye usually runs its course in seven to ten days; it will not respond to antibiotic treatment.

Bacterial conjunctivitis will produce abundant thick yellow or green discharge from the eye. Your little girl might complain of eye pain and her eye or eyelid might appear swollen. The doctor will prescribe an antibiotic for bacterial conjunctivitis. Once treatment begins, the symptoms should be under control within five days.

Allergic conjunctivitis is pinkeye that accompanies allergies. Unlike viral and bacterial conjunctivitis, allergic conjunctivitis is not contagious. Both eyes are usually red, teary, and itchy. Other allergy symptoms are usually present as well: sneezing, itchy nose with watery nasal discharge, and scratchy throat. Seasonal allergies, pollen, animal dander, and dust are the typical causes of allergic conjunctivitis.

Is my newborn's watery eye conjunctivitis?

It's not uncommon for an infant to be born with a partially blocked tear duct, a condition called *nasolacrimal duct obstruction.* That blockage produces continuous tearing from the inner corner of the eye, mucous drainage from the eye, and crusting over the eyelashes. Most of the time the blockage opens on it's own within several months.

You can help to open a blocked tear duct with a very gentle massage of the duct area 3 to 4 times a day. With the pad of a clean fingertip—one that has a very short nail—gently massage the area between the inner corner of the eye and the bridge of the nose. Make eight to ten tiny circles each time you work on the area—use a gentle but firm touch. This attentive touch is all that is needed to help open the duct.

How can you help . . .

. . . keep her comfortable

Clean her eyes a couple of times during the day with a clean soft cloth that is moistened with warm water. (If your child has *allergic* conjunctivitis, use a cool compress to soothe her eyes.) Have her close both her eyes, or one at a time, if that's easier for her to tolerate. Pass the cloth over her closed eye, moving from the inside of the eye toward the outside. Use a clean area of the cloth for each pass over her eye. You'll want to do this in the morning when she wakes up to "unstick" her eyes. Replace the cloth after each use to avoid reinfecting her eye. If you are using a bowl of warm water to compress her eyes, make sure you don't dip the part of the cloth you used on her eyes back into the water bowl. "Double dipping" can contaminate the water.

Discourage your child from rubbing her eyes, even if they are irritated and bothering her. Use a warm compress to help soothe and clear her eyes. You can use either warm water or warm eyebright tea to compress her eyes. The herb eyebright helps to relieve swelling and inflammation of the eyes. Steep one teaspoon or two teabags of eyebright in 8 ounces of warm water for 5 to 7 minutes. Use the warm tea to compress her eyes for 10 minutes at a time once or twice a day. Again, be careful not to "double dip."

Encourage your little girl to limit the time she spends watching television and playing on the computer or with video games. Activities that don't involve focused eye involvement, such as listening to music or playing with toys, will be easier on her sore eyes.

Keep your child home from childcare or school until the symptoms of infectious conjunctivitis have cleared up. A few days at home might prevent your child from getting sicker and from passing this infection on to others. If your child is older and has many after-school activities, allow her to skip them while she's contagious.

If you are letting her stay home from school, keep her in an area where the temperature is warm and stable and where the lighting is not too bright. Let her rest. Rest and sleep are the greatest healers. The body knows it; use its wisdom to your advantage.

. . . prevent conjunctivitis

Make sure to wash your hands regularly, and teach your children to wash theirs, particularly after being in contact with anyone who might be sick. Using soap and warm water or an alcohol-based hand rub (anti-bacterial products aren't necessary) is the easiest way to prevent the spread of disease. Hand-to-hand contact and contact with infected objects is the source of many ailments, including conjunctivitis.

Try to encourage your child to avoid touching her eyes. If she does touch her face or eyes, have her wash her hands or use an alcohol-based hand rub afterward.

Wash bed linens and towels regularly, and avoid sharing towels and linens with others in the household.

Try to avoid coming into close contact with another child who has conjunctivitis.

A word on diet

Modifying your child's diet will help her to recover quickly. Dairy products tend to increase the body's production of mucus, so avoid giving her any cow's milk or milk products. This includes cheeses, yogurt, cottage cheese, ice cream, and puddings. You can try substituting soy milk and soy-based cheeses.

Increasing fluids helps to thin mucous secretions—water, diluted juices, clear broths, and diluted herb teas are good choices. You can even offer her eyebright tea to drink. Steamed and fresh fruits and vegetables and lightly prepared chicken and fish are easy to digest when you're fighting an infection.

Avoid high fat foods, fried foods, or processed or fatty meats, which are often difficult to digest.

And, as always, keep her away from highly processed foods: white sugar (candy, cookies, pastries, sodas), white flour and bread products, and foods with chemicals and preservatives.

Treatment

The areas and points that are used in this treatment are aimed at soothing and reducing inflammation in and around the eyes. Some points are used to strengthen the system. Use this treatment if your child has conjunctivitis; it can also be used to soothe eyestrain or eye soreness. If your child has cold symptoms along with conjunctivitis, use the points on page XX [X-Ref] to help her heal from that as well.

All of the shaded areas in the treatment illustrations are useful in helping your child to feel better. Some areas are shaded lightly, others somewhat darker. The lightly shaded areas need the least amount of work; the darkest areas need the most attention. Work on the lightly shaded areas just once or twice during the course of the treatment; work on the darker areas more frequently, staying at each area no more than 3 to 5 seconds at a time. When you treat an older child, adolescent, or adult, you can locate the acupoints within the darkly shaded areas. But when you treat a baby or young child, working generally in the area of an acupoint will produce the desired result.

Use a gentle touch when you massage your child. When you are working on a baby, all the pressure that's needed is the degree of pressure you would use if you were finger painting or checking to see if a cake is finished baking.

The best time to work on your child is any time she's open to it. Take your time; make her comfortable; relax.

1. Begin with a massage of the forehead on and above the eyebrows. Stroke from the bridge of the nose across the eyebrows and out toward the temples.

2. Massage the upper portion of the cheekbones, starting at the nose and ending at the temples.

   Massage of forehead and cheekbones will soothe any muscular tension that accompanies conjunctivitis. It will help to reduce swelling and increase lymphatic drainage in the area.

3. Gently press the point that lies above the bridge of the nose in between the eyebrows.

   Extra point Yintang is used in the treatment of ailments of the eye.

4. Gently press the point that lies between the bridge of the nose and the inside edge of the eye.

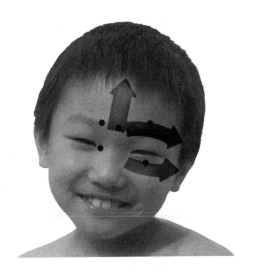

Treatment areas of the face for conjunctivitis

Bladder 1 is used in the treatment of eye ailments. The nasolacrimal duct lies slightly below Bladder 1.

5. Gently press the inside edge of the eyebrow.

   Bladder 2 is used in the treatment of eye ailments.

6. Press the point that lies on the forehead just above the midpoint of the eyebrow.

   Gall Bladder 14 is used in the treatment of eye ailments and headache.

7. Press the point that lies on the temple midway between the outer edge of the eyebrow and the outer edge of the eye.

   Extra point Taiyang is used in the treatment of eye ailments and headache.

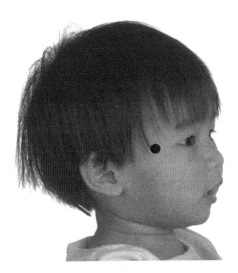

Temple acupoint associated with the treatment of conjunctivitis

8. Gently press the point that lies beneath the eye on the uppermost part of the cheekbone.

   Stomach 1 is used in the treatment of eye ailments.

9. Work on the backside of the hand between the index finger and the thumb.

   Colon 4 works to strengthen immune function.

10. Gently massage the outside of the lower leg, giving a bit more attention to the area just beneath the knee.

    Stomach 36 works with Spleen 6 to help strengthen immune function.

11. Massage the inside of the lower leg several inches above the anklebone.

    Spleen 6 works with Stomach 36 to help strengthen immune function.

12. Massage the space between the long bones of the big toe and the second toe.

    Liver 2, closest to the toe, helps to reduce inflammation; Liver 3, closer to the foot, is used in the treatment of the eye.

13. Gently massage the outside of the pinky toe.

    Bladder 65, 66, and 67 are used to treat ailments of the eye and headache.

14. Gently massage the back of the neck starting at the base of the skull, moving down the neck toward the shoulders and across the upper shoulders.

    The release of the upper trapezius muscle will help soften the musculature of the neck and shoulders. Massage of this area will also assist with lymphatic drainage of the head and neck. Each of the yang meridians travels through this area. Its release contributes to the free flow of energy through the system.

15. Gently stroke the back, alongside the spine, down toward the pelvis.

    Massage of this area simply feels good and will help make your child feel better all the way around.

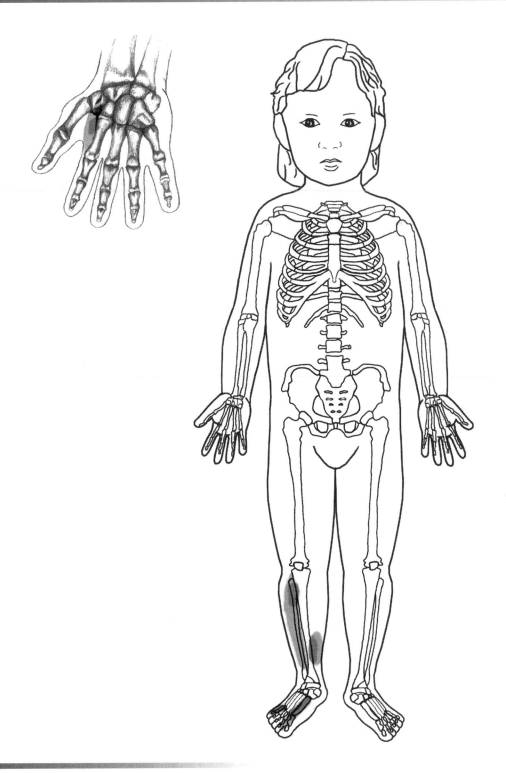

Treatment areas of the lower leg, back,
and hand for conjunctivitis

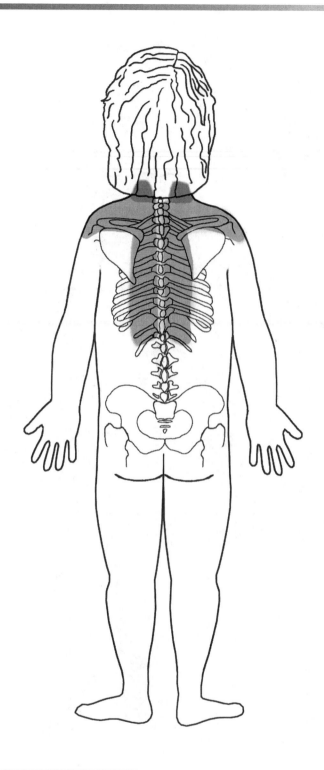

Treatment areas of the back for
conjunctivitis

Fever

When should you check with your doctor?

Check with your doctor if an infant of three months or younger has a fever of 100.4° F or higher. If your baby is between three and six months old and has a fever of 101° F or higher, or if he is between six and twenty-four months and has a fever of 102° F or higher, check with your doctor.*

If your child is two years or older, call your doctor if his fever lasts longer than three days; if he is younger than two, call your doctor if the fever lasts longer than twenty-four to thirty-six hours.

Call your doctor if your child is listless, irritable, or unresponsive; is crying weakly or uncontrollably; has difficulty breathing or swallowing; if he has a severe headache or stomachache; is vomiting; has diarrhea, or pain when he urinates; if he has an unusual rash; or if you believe he may be dehydrated (see page XX [[diarrhea]]).

Call your doctor if your child has had a seizure.

Febrile seizures

A small percentage of children will occasionally have a convulsion or seizure as a result of a rapid increase in body temperature. Febrile seizures can be terrifying to

*Temperature ranges here refer to a temperature taken rectally. A temperature taken orally is approximately 1 degree lower than a temperature taken rectally. A digital rectal thermometer is recommended for children younger than 3 months. Electronic ear thermometers are accurate when used with children over the age of 3 months.

a parent, but they generally don't harm the child. When your child has a febrile seizure he will begin to twitch and his arms and legs may flail; his eyes may roll back and he may lose consciousness. When the seizure is over he will likely be very tired and want to sleep.

Try to stay calm if your child has a seizure. It's usually over within minutes. Let your doctor know as soon as possible if your child has had a febrile seizure. If your child has a seizure lasting ten minutes or longer, call for emergency help.

What is it?

Body temperature varies throughout the day, depending on the activities that you're engaged in, how you're dressed, and the time of day. It will be at its highest in the late afternoon and evening. Normal body temperature, taken rectally, is considered to be 98.6° F (37° C). Temperature taken orally is usually one degree Fahrenheit lower than temperature taken rectally.

A fever is an elevated body temperature. Most of the time it's the body's way of fighting off an infection. Often parents, especially new parents, become upset when they see that their little one has a fever (especially the new baby's first fever)—but it's important to remember that fever is an indication that the body's defenses are working as they should.

When the immune system begins to fight infection, the body's temperature goes higher than its norm. Metabolism, breathing, and heart rate are increased, along with the production of white blood cells and antibodies. Along with a fever there might be chills, headache, weakness, and lack of appetite. Sweating is the first sign that the body's temperature is starting to return to the normal range. It's the body's way of dispersing excess heat.

Because a fever is the body's way of fighting infection, it isn't necessary to treat most low-grade fevers (those ranging from 100–102° F) to bring them down. Fevers ranging from 102–104° F are considered moderate fevers that are beneficial to the healing process. They can be treated with fever-reducing medications such as ibuprofen or acetaminophen if your child is uncomfortable. Fevers that are higher than 104° F may be making your child uncomfortable; most doctors recommend that steps be taken to reduce, but not eliminate, the fever. Check with your doctor if you are unsure about whether to give your child medication to bring down a fever, or how much to give him.

Your child's behavior, rather than his temperature, is a fairly good indication of how sick he is. Some kids can tolerate a fever of 103°F and still be playful, alert, and happy. Other kids will be cranky or sleepy and reluctant to eat with a fever of 101° F. Most of the time you know how sick your child is just by looking at him. When your usually unstoppable four year old only wants to be held and cuddled, regardless of the number on the thermometer, you know he's sick.

Should I give him fever-reducing medications?

Non steroidal anti-inflammatory drugs (NSAIDS), such as ibuprofen and acetaminophen, are sometimes the first thing we think of when our child has a fever. But remember that temperature fluctuates through the day, and when we're sick sometimes our bodies need that bit of fever to heal. Use medications cautiously when you need to, and only use them when they're needed the most.

What causes it?

Fever is not a disease in and of itself: it is caused by the presence of an infection. A viral infection is the most common reason that children develop fevers. The fever that accompanies most viral infections can be expected to last two to three days with a temperature range of 101–103° F. Fever of 104° F or higher is more likely to be related to a bacterial infection, such as a sinus infection, a urinary tract infection, or strep throat. If your child's fever is 104° F or higher, he should be seen by a medical doctor so that the source of his infection can be determined and the infection can be treated as needed.

How you can help . . .

. . . keep him comfortable

Avoid overdressing him. A single layer of light clothing or pajamas and a light blanket for a bedcover, is generally all he'll need to stay comfortable. Keep him in a room or an area of the house where the temperature is stable and warm.

If his fever is higher than 102° F, try giving him a sponge bath using lukewarm water to help bring it down. Avoid using alcohol—it will cool the skin too quickly, which can lead to the shivers as the body tries to reheat itself. If your child is old enough, let him relax in a warm bath for 10 minutes or so. Stay with him to make sure that he doesn't get chilled.

Encourage him to rest. Rest and sleep are the body's way of healing itself. Keep him home from school until his temperature has remained in the normal range for twenty-four hours. It's not uncommon to wake up in the morning with a normal temperature and feeling well, only to find that the fever has returned late in the day. Make sure that your child is truly well before he returns to school and after-school activities.

If your child is particularly uncomfortable or has a fever of over 102° F, speak to your doctor about giving him acetaminophen (Tylenol) or ibuprofen (Advil). Avoid using aspirin with children. It may cause Reye's syndrome, a rare but potentially harmful disease.

. . . prevent him from getting sick

The simplest way to avoid getting sick is to make sure to wash your hands regularly and to teach your children to wash theirs. Using soap and warm water or an alcohol-based hand rub (anti-bacterials aren't necessary) is the easiest way to prevent the spread of disease. Colds, the flu, and many other diseases are caused by hand-to-hand contact. Teach your kids to wash after they've touched their face, coughed, or sneezed into their hand or blown their nose. Spreading an infection can be prevented if a child gets into the habit of washing his hands before he eats, after he's used the bathroom, when he comes in from playing outdoors, after he's played with or touched the family pet, and after he's been with someone who is sick or has a cold. Little things can make the biggest difference.

Teach your children to use tissues to cover mouth and nose when coughing or sneezing. Throw the tissues away immediately.

If tissues aren't available, teach your children to sneeze or cough into the crook of the arm (the bend in the elbow) rather than into the hand. Not only will droplets be prevented from pouring into the air, but there is less of a possibility that they will contaminate objects by touching them with their hands.

Try to encourage your children to keep their hands, toys, pencils, and anything else that isn't food out of their mouths. Wash toys and other objects frequently to prevent them from being the source of disease.

Avoid sharing drinking glasses, eating utensils, and towels when someone is sick. Wash or change drinking glasses (particularly those used in the bathroom) after each use. Replace your child's toothbrush after he's recovered.

A word on diet

It's very important to keep your child's fluid intake high while he has a fever in order to avoid dehydration. He may not want to eat, and that's okay. But you should try to get him to drink. Sipping purified water, diluted juices, broths, herbal teas, or oral rehydration fluids throughout the day will help to keep him well hydrated. Freshly squeezed grapefruit juice and orange juice are ideal. You can offer him frozen juice pops if he's unwilling to sip fluids.

If your child wants to eat, offer him foods that are easy to digest: steamed and fresh fruits and vegetables, eggs, and lightly prepared chicken and fish. Chicken soup is a very good choice.

Treatment

This treatment can be used whenever your child has a fever. If he has other symptoms, such as a sore throat or cough, you can use the treatment for that particular condition and add these points to it. You'll end up treating his ailment as well as his fever.

All of the shaded areas in the treatment illustrations are useful in helping your child to feel better. Some areas are shaded lightly, others somewhat darker. The lightly shaded areas need the least amount of work; the darkest areas need the most attention. Work on the lightly shaded areas just once or twice during the course of the treatment; work on the darker areas more frequently, staying at each area no more than 3 to 5 seconds at a time. When you treat an older child, adolescent, or adult, you can locate the acupoints within the darkly shaded areas. But when you treat a baby or young child, working generally in the area of an acupoint will produce the desired result.

Use a gentle touch when you massage your child. When you are working on a baby, all the pressure that's needed is the degree of pressure you would use if you were finger painting or checking to see if a cake is finished baking.

The best time to work on your child is any time he's open to it. Take your time; make him comfortable. Both of you can relax while you help him feel better.

1. Gently massage down the front of the body, starting at the breastbone and working down toward the belly.

2. Gently stroke the upper chest. Start at the breastbone and work out toward the area where the arms meet the body.

   Working on this area will help to relax him and open the chest. Pectoralis major lies across the top of the chest. Massage here will help ease breathing.

3. Gently massage the outside of the back of the arm, beginning at the upper shoulder, working down toward the elbow and then to the hand.

   Massage here follows the course of the Colon channel.

4. Massage the area that lies on the outside of the elbow, at the place where the elbow creases when you bend the arm.

   Colon 11 is used to treat inflammation and fever.

5. Massage the back side of the index finger, starting at the fleshy part between the thumb and the index finger and working down to the nail.

   Colon 1 and Colon 2 are used to treat fevers. Colon 4 is used to strengthen immune function. Colon 4 is used with Liver 3 to calm the system.

6. Massage the inside of the lower arm just above the wrist.

   Pericardium 6 is used to treat fevers.

7. Massage the palm side of the middle finger, focusing the greatest attention at the tip of the middle finger.

   Pericardium 9 is used to treat fevers.

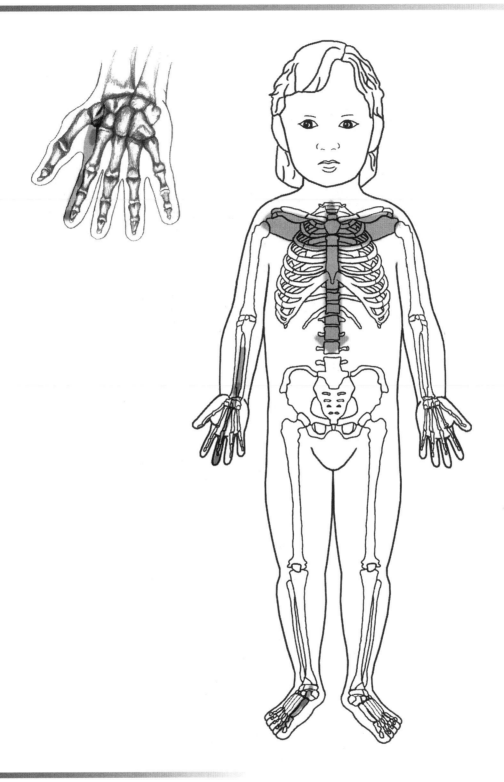

*Treatment areas on the front and
hand for fever*

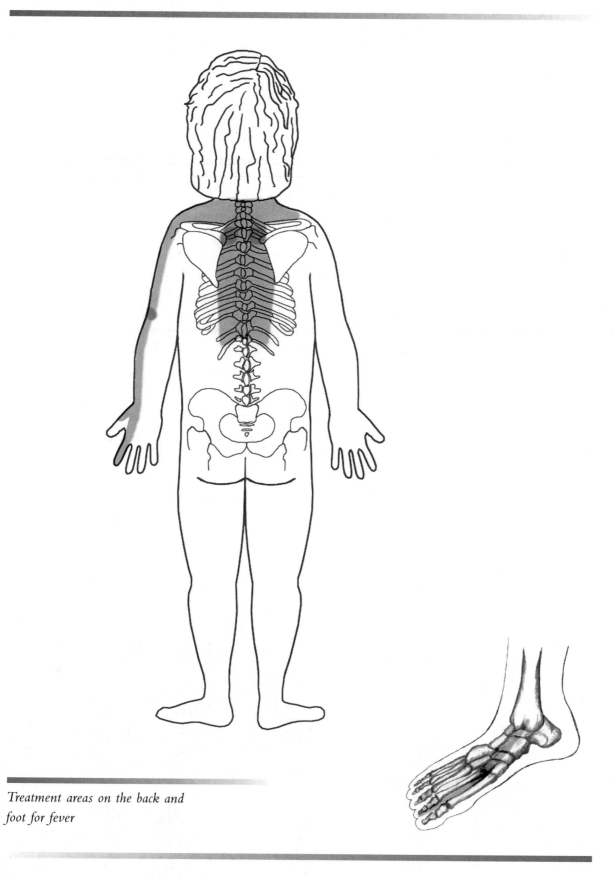

*Treatment areas on the back and
foot for fever*

8. Massage the area between the big toe and the second toe, focusing the greatest attention at the place where the bones of the big toe and second toe meet at the foot.

   Liver 3 is used with Colon 4 to calm the system.

9. Massage the center of the upper back, particularly the area that is in line with the top of the shoulder blades.

   Bladder 13, which lies between the top of the shoulder blade and the spine, is used in the treatment of fevers.

10. Gently stroke the back, alongside the spine, down toward the pelvis.

    Massage of this area simply feels good and will help soothe your child and make him feel better all the way around.

Constipation and Gas

When should you check with your doctor?

Check with your doctor if your baby or child has constipation lasting for more than three or four days, if he has recurrent or persistent constipation, or if constipation is accompanied by vomiting or the unwillingness to eat, or if there is blood or mucus in his stools or a cut or tear in his rectum.

What is it?

Constipation is a change in bowel habits. Each child's bowel habits are different, and every attentive parent knows just what their child's bowel habits are. On average, babies have four bowel movements a day. Some babies have as few as one bowel movement every third or fourth day; they're comfortable, they're happy, and they're eating. But if they haven't moved their bowels by the fifth day, it's likely that they are constipated.

By two years old the child may only have two bowel movements each day, and by the time your child is four he's probably only having one bowel movement a day, much like the usual adult rhythm. If your child doesn't move his bowels for four or five days, or if his stool is hard and dry or resembles pellets or little dry balls, he is probably constipated. If he's constipated he may have a stomachache or pain while trying to pass stools.

Constipation is more common in formula-fed babies than in

breastfed babies. Because breast milk digests so readily, it's not uncommon for a breastfed baby to go without a bowel movement for as long as a week. If your baby is breastfed and does not move his bowels for several days but seems to be comfortable and is eating normally, he's probably fine.

What causes it?

The most common cause of constipation in babies and children is not having enough fluid and fiber in their diet. The fiber in your baby's diet and the fluid he takes in combine to form his stool. Insufficient fiber causes the stool to be too soft to move through the system well; insufficient fluid will lead to hard and dry stool that is difficult to pass.

If your baby is still on formula, it may contain too few carbohydrates and too much fat for stool formation and elimination. Check with your doctor if you have a question about the baby's formula.

If your older child is constipated he may be drinking too much cow's milk. If he's is drinking more than 12 to 16 ounces of cow's milk daily, it may be a bit too much for his system.

If your child is eating solid foods, he may not have enough fiber in his diet. Highly processed foods, foods that are high in white flour and white sugar, and excessive amounts of cow's milk products (cheese, yogurt, puddings, and ice cream) may be the culprits. All are low in fiber and may contribute to his constipation.

Chronic constipation occurs frequently between the ages of two and four, the time of potty training. If the child has ever been constipated he may remember the discomfort of trying to pass dry stools and may willfully prevent himself from moving his bowels. This may be the beginning of a vicious cycle leading to chronic constipation.

How you can help

If your baby or young child is constipated, offer him diluted prune or apple juice or apricot nectar. One ounce of juice diluted with three ounces of purified water helps to get things moving.

If your little one is constipated and is having difficulty or pain when he tries to move his bowels, you may consider using a glycerine suppository or an enema formulated specifically for infants and children. (Glycerine is a food, not a medication, and is safe to use with your baby.) Glycerine melts in the rectum, and the resultant stimulation leads to a bowel movement.

Make sure that your child is drinking ample fluids on a daily basis, especially purified water. You can give an infant 2 to 4 ounces of water during the day. Older babies and children would benefit from drinking 8 to 12 ounces of purified water throughout the course of the day. If you introduce purified water to your child when he is a baby, it's likely that that he'll be willing to drink water rather than sweetened beverages when he is older.

If your baby is taking a cow's milk formula and he tends toward constipation, talk to your doctor about trying a different formulation or a soy-based formula as a replacement.

Keep an ample amount of fiber in the diet of babies over four months of age who are eating solid foods. Fruits such as apples, plums, prunes, and pears, raw or cooked vegetables, and whole-grain cereals such as oatmeal, brown rice, and bran cereals are all good sources of fiber. Taken daily, a small amount of yogurt with active cultures is beneficial for digestion and elimination.

Keep the amount of bananas, white rice and rice cereals, cow's milk and dairy products, and highly processed foods containing white flour and white sugar to a minimum in your older child's diet.

Treatment

Use the following treatment any time your child is constipated, when he's uncomfortable because he has lower belly gas, or to help your child's digestion to stay healthy and regular.

All of the shaded areas in the treatment illustrations are useful in helping your child to move his bowels. Some areas are shaded lightly, others somewhat darker. The lightly shaded areas need the least amount of work; the darkest areas need the most attention. Work on the lightly shaded areas just once or twice during the course of the treatment; work on the darker areas more frequently, staying at each area no more than 3 to 5 seconds at a time. When you treat an older child, adolescent, or adult, you can locate the acupoints within the darkly shaded areas. But when you treat a baby or young child, working generally in the area of an acupoint will produce the desired result.

Use a gentle touch when you massage your child. When you are working on a baby, all the pressure that's needed is the degree of pressure you would use if you were finger painting or checking to see if a cake is finished baking. This can be fun and pleasurable for both of you. Talk to you child when you work on him. It can be a really good experience for you, too. Treatment time combines the joy of connecting with your little one with the pleasure in being able to actively do something that will help him be happier, healthier and more comfortable.

1. Begin with a gentle massage of your child's stomach and abdomen, beginning at the ribcage and working down toward the lower belly. Repeat 2 to 3 times.

2. Gently massage the lower belly, beginning on the right side by the hipbone. Work up the right side, then work across the belly above the belly button, and then move down the belly toward the left hipbone.

   The course of this massage stroke follows the direction of the colon: up the ascending colon on the right side of the body, across the transverse colon just above the navel, and down the descending colon on the left side of the body. In working in this way you are stimulating the movement of gas and fecal matter through the colon toward the rectum, where it will be eliminated.

3. Gently press the point that lies at the midpoint between the break in the ribcage and the belly button.

   Conception Vessel 12 regulates digestion.

4. Gently press the point that lies at the midpoint between Conception Vessel 12 and the belly button.

   Conception Vessel 10 stimulates digestion.

5. Gently press the point that lies approximately 1 inch below the belly button.

   Conception Vessel 6 stimulates elimination.

6. Gently press the area a couple of inches to the side of the belly button on both sides.

   Stomach 25 helps to alleviate constipation and stomachache.

7. Massage the outside of the lower leg from the knee to the ankle. Give a bit more attention to the area a couple of inches below the knee.

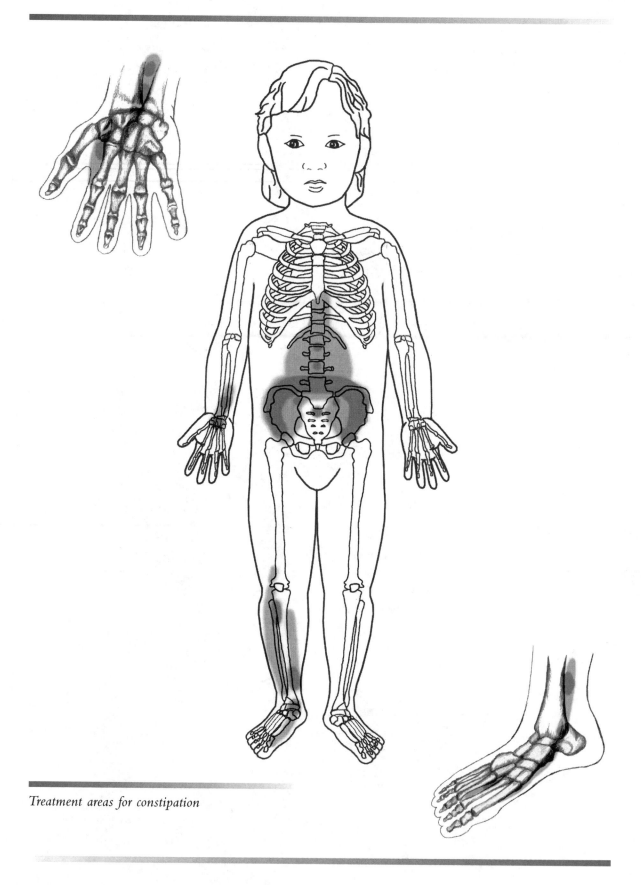

Treatment areas for constipation

The Stomach meridian lies on the outside of the lower leg. Stomach 36 tones all aspects of digestion and elimination. Stomach 36 works with Spleen 6 to strengthen immune function.

8. Gently massage the inside of the lower leg a couple of inches above the inside anklebone.

   Spleen 6 aids in digestion and elimination. Spleen 6 works with Stomach 36 to strengthen immune function.

9. Gently massage the top of the inner ankle.

   Spleen 5 helps to balance the digestive system.

10. Gently massage between the long bones leading up to the second and third toes.

    Stomach 43 helps to reduce abdominal pain.

11. Gently massage the back of the wrist, 1 inch or so above the wrist fold.

    Triple Warmer 6 helps to alleviate constipation. Triple Warmer 5 works with Triple Warmer 6 and Pericardium 7 to alleviate pain associated with constipation.

12. Gently massage the front of the wrist 1inch or so above the wrist fold.

    Pericardium 7 works with Triple Warmer 5 and Triple Warmer 6 to alleviate pain associated with constipation.

13. Gently massage the web between the thumb and the index finger.

    Colon 4 helps to alleviate constipation.

14. Press gently into the small of the lower back, where the spine meets the pelvis.

    Bladder 25 is used in the treatment of constipation.

15. Massage the sacrum, the flat bone that lies at the bottom of the spine and joins the pelvis at its center.

    Bladder 34 is used in the treatment of constipation.

16. Gently massage the muscles lying beside the spine, the buttocks, and the backs of the thighs.

    Massage here will promote relaxation, helping to calm and soothe.

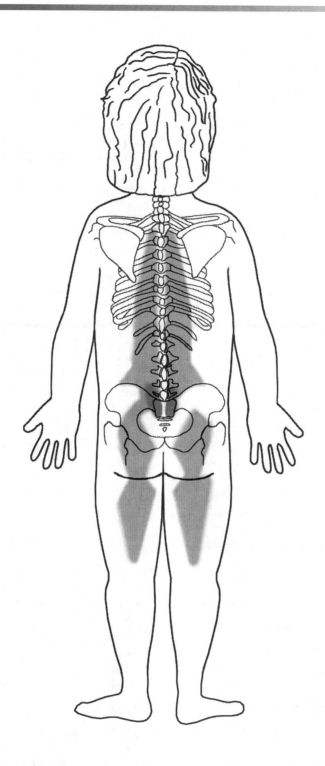

Treatment areas for constipation

Diarrhea

When should you check with your doctor?

If your newborn or your baby younger than four months develops diarrhea, check with your doctor. If diarrhea lasts longer than forty-eight hours in your older child, or is accompanied by vomiting or a fever of 101.5° F or higher or blood in the stool, consult with your physician.

Long-term diarrhea, lasting for longer than two weeks, can be a sign of a more serious intestinal disease or functional problem and should be evaluated by a physician.

Dehydration in an infant or child is a serious problem that must be addressed promptly. A child who is crying without producing tears, has not urinated for three hours or more, has a dry or sticky mouth and tongue, and is listless and irritable or who has the appearance of a sunken abdomen, eyes, cheeks, or fontanel may be dehydrated. If your child has any of the symptoms of dehydration, contact your physician immediately.

What is dehydration?

Dehydration can be a very serious problem for children and adults alike, but especially for an infant or young child. A body is dehydrated when it doesn't have the amount water and fluid it needs to function properly. We can become dehydrated when the amount of fluid that we lose is more than we take in. We lose fluids rapidly through vomiting, diarrhea, fever, heavy sweating, and excessive urination. It's difficult to keep fluid levels up when we're sick. For many of us it is exactly when we have diarrhea or we're vomiting that we don't want to drink anything. But that is exactly when we *must* drink fluids.

If you or your child has diarrhea, is vomiting, or has a fever, sip water, diluted juices, and broths throughout the day. You can offer your child oral rehydration fluids such as Pedialyte. Make sure that your child is urinating regularly, has a moist mouth, and is producing tears. Keep a close eye on your child if she's sick; keep the potential for dehydration in mind and do what you can to avoid it. If your child is sick and you believe that she hasn't been taking in the fluids she needs, discuss it with your physician.

What is it?

Diarrhea is loose or watery stools that occur more than three times a day. Diarrhea is fairly common in children and will often clear up on its own in a day or so. If your child has diarrhea, in addition to loose and frequent bowel movements she may experience cramping and abdominal pain, particularly just before a bowel movement. Bloating, nausea, urgency, lack of bowel control, fever, and bloody stools might also accompany diarrhea.

Diarrhea may cause considerable fluid loss very quickly, and a child with diarrhea must be watched carefully for signs of dehydration, a serious problem for an infant or young child.

What causes it?

A baby or child can develop diarrhea from something as simple as a change in formula, the introduction of a new food, a reaction to an antibiotic, or even teething. Diarrhea caused by something like this is generally very short-lived.

If your child's diarrhea is from a virus or bacteria, she's likely to feel mildly feverish and may be vomiting as well. Diarrhea that is caused by a bacterial or viral infection will usually last for two or three days, although it may cause occasional bouts of diarrhea for up to two weeks.

Food allergies or intolerances may cause cramping and diarrhea following each meal. If this is happening to your child, try eliminating milk and milk products first to see how she reacts; milk allergies are very common in children. Other frequent sources of food allergies are wheat, soy, eggs, peanuts, and tree nuts. Try eliminating them if need be. If the cramping and diarrhea continue, talk with your doctor about changing your child's diet.

Healthy toddlers may develop diarrhea from drinking too much juice or too many sweetened drinks. If your child has diarrhea but it otherwise thriving, ask yourself if she's been consuming too many sugar-laden beverages. It's generally recommended that young children have no more than 4 to 6 ounces of undiluted juice daily because of its high sugar content.

Eating tainted food produces a short-lived but intense period of diarrhea and possibly vomiting. In some cases a low-grade fever might be present as well.

Other causes of diarrhea include parasites, intestinal disease, or functional bowel problems. These would likely cause diarrhea that would last for an extended period of time. If your child has bouts of diarrhea for more than two weeks she should be seen by a physician so the source can be determined.

What is the rotavirus?

The leading cause of acute gastroenteritis in infants and children is the *rotavirus*. Sometimes referred to as the "stomach flu" or a "stomach virus," rotavirus causes severe diarrhea. Rotavirus is highly contagious. Many children will become infected with it by the age of five. It is most commonly experienced in the winter and spring months, and it is one of the five most common illnesses that keep kids from going to school (along with the common cold, ear infections, conjunctivitis, and sore throat). Children between the ages of four and twenty-four months are at the greatest risk of being exposed to the rotavirus, particularly those who attend daycare. The rotavirus is passed from person to person through contact with the feces of an infected child. Unfortunately the virus is present in the stool of an infected person days before symptoms begin, and can persist for up to ten days after symptoms cease.

Hand washing is essential to preventing the spread of rotavirus. It is particularly important to wash your hands carefully after handling diapers, using the toilet, or helping a child to use the toilet. The virus remains active on objects that are touched with infected hands; it can easily be passed to another in this way. The virus can also be passed to another through droplets of saliva and mucus that are sneezed or coughed into the air.

Rotavirus infection usually begins with a fever, vomiting, and a stomachache. Diarrhea soon follows, and that may last between three and five days. Symptoms range from mild to severe. Just as with diarrhea from any other source, fluid loss and dehydration is the greatest concern with a child who is infected with rotavirus. Your child must be watched carefully to prevent dehydration.

How you can help . . .

. . . keep her comfortable

The most important thing that you can do for your child is to replenish the fluids that are lost through diarrhea. Encourage her to drink at least a small amount of fluid every hour, anywhere from 1 to 2 teaspoons to 2 ounces. Nursing mothers should continue to nurse. Your formula-fed baby might have some difficulty digesting a cow's milk formula while she has diarrhea, so you might consider switching to a formula that is soy based. You can offer your baby oral rehydration fluids, such as Pedialyte, Ceralyte, or Infalyte. Offer the older child water, broths, soups, herbal teas, or rehydration fluids. Try to avoid giving her fruit juices or other sweetened beverages, which may make her diarrhea worse.

It's very important to keep your baby's bottom clean. The enzymes passed in diarrhea can wreak havoc on your little one's delicate skin. It won't be enough to use only a premoistened wipe when you change her diaper. Wash your baby's bottom with warm water and use a protective lotion or cream to protect that delicate skin. Could there be anything more uncomfortable than to have diarrhea and an irritated bottom at the same time?

. . . prevent the spread of diarrhea

Keep your hands and changing areas clean. Wash your hands well after handling soiled diapers and changing your baby. Dispose of soiled diapers promptly and carefully.

Teach your older children the importance of washing their hands or using an alcohol-based hand rub after using the bathroom and before eating. Hand washing is the easiest way to prevent the spread of disease.

Make sure that your child's toys remain clean by washing them periodically, especially if your child is at that stage where everything goes in her mouth.

Replace your kitchen sponges frequently. Used sponges have been found to be a major breeding ground for bacteria within the kitchen.

A Word on Diet

Some experts recommend the BRAT diet—bananas, rice, applesauce, and toast—to help bind the bowel of a child who is old enough to eat solid foods. Others believe that it is important to allow the child to eat what she feels comfortable with. Most agree, however, that dairy products and sugary foods and drinks (as well as those containing artificial sweeteners such as sorbitol and saccharin) and carbonated beverages can make diarrhea worse and should be avoided. See what foods work best for your child. The key here is to remember what you felt like when you've had diarrhea. If you were hungry you could eat. But sometimes you were nauseous and could not. Watch your child, see how she feels, and approach her from that point of view. Remember that it's more important that she drink than eat.

Treatment

You can help ease your child's discomfort using this treatment. The best time to work on your child is after she's had a bowel movement and she's all cleaned up, although you can work on her any time she's open to it.

All of the shaded areas in the treatment illustrations are useful in helping your child to feel better. Some areas are shaded lightly, others somewhat darker. The lightly shaded areas need the least amount of work; the darkest areas need the most attention. Work on the lightly shaded areas just once or twice during the course of the treatment;

work on the darker areas more frequently, staying at each area no more than 3 to 5 seconds at a time. When you treat an older child, adolescent, or adult, you can locate the acupoints within the darkly shaded areas. But when you treat a baby or young child, working generally in the area of an acupoint will produce the desired result.

Use a gentle touch when you massage your child. When you are working on a baby, all the pressure that's needed is the degree of pressure you would use if you were finger painting or using an internal mouse pad on a laptop computer.

Take your time; make her comfortable; relax.

1. Gently massage the upper chest, beginning at the breastbone and moving downward to the upper belly.

   Treatment here brings energy down from the chest and into the belly.

2. Gently press the point that lies at the midpoint between the break in the ribcage and the belly button.

   Conception Vessel 12 regulates digestion.

3. Gently press the area a couple of inches to the side of the belly button on both sides.

   Stomach 25 works with Stomach 37 to alleviate stomachache and diarrhea.

4. Gently press the area about one-quarter of the way down the outside of the lower leg.

   The Stomach meridian lies on the outside of the lower leg. Stomach 37 works with Stomach 25 to help to alleviate stomachache and diarrhea.

5. Gently massage the inside of the ankle on the top of the foot.
   Spleen 5 helps to balance the digestive system.

6. Gently massage the palm side of the index fingers, middle fingers, ring fingers, and pinkies.

   These points help to calm indigestion in children.

7. Massage the lower back moving down toward the upper part of the pelvis and the sacrum, the flat bone that lies at the bottom of the spine.

   Bladder 25, 26, and 28 work to alleviate stomachache and calm diarrhea.

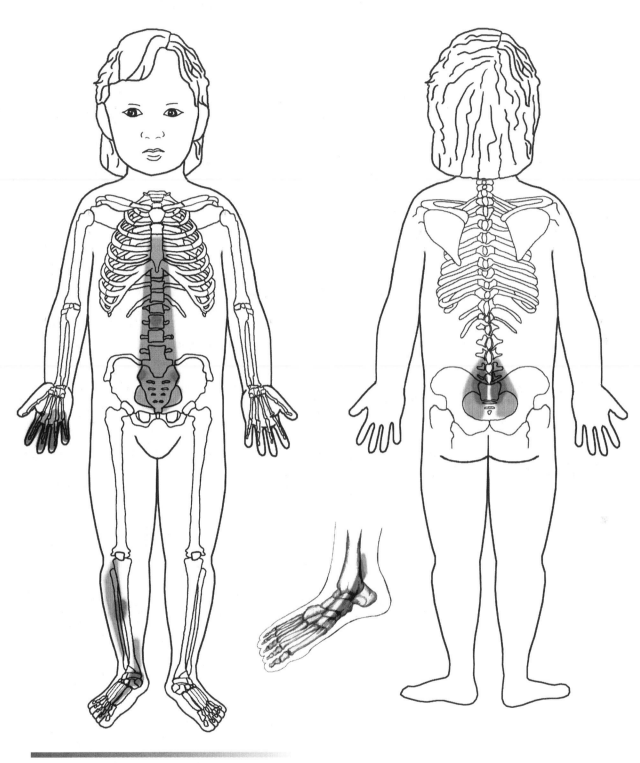

*Treatment areas of the front,
back, and hand for diarrhea*

Vomiting

When should you check with your doctor?

Check with your physician if your child is vomiting for four to six hours continuously, repeatedly vomiting for a twenty-four-hour period of time, is forcefully vomiting a great distance from his body (projectile vomiting), or if there is blood or bright green or yellow fluid in the vomit. If vomiting starts shortly after a head injury, call your doctor.

Dehydration (page XX [X-Ref]) is a very serious problem in infants and children. It can result from repeated or continuous vomiting commonly experienced with a stomach flu. If your child appears to have any of the symptoms of dehydration, consult with your physician immediately. Those symptoms of dehydration are crying without producing tears, not urinating for three hours or more, a dry or sticky mouth and tongue, fever greater than 101.5° F, listlessness and irritability, or the appearance of a sunken abdomen, eyes, cheeks or fontanel.

What is it?

Vomiting is unpleasant, at best. It's the forceful passing of partially digested food through the mouth. Most of the time vomiting is associated with nausea and diarrhea and may begin with lack of appetite, queasiness, burping, and nausea. There may be pain or aching in the upper stomach, along with increased salivation. The total picture is one in which the person who is vomiting is uncomfortable and unhappy, regardless of size and age.

Is spitting up the same as vomiting?

Vomiting is very different from "spitting up." When food is vomited, it has already been partially digested. Milk will be curdled and food will be broken down by the stomach's digestive enzymes. You'll clearly detect a sour odor in the food that has been brought up.

When a baby spits up, the milk that went into his mouth returns without being changed very much. There is little or no odor. He may be spitting up milk along with air when you've burped him, or he may be spitting up because he's eaten too much.

As many as 50 percent of all infants younger than six months old spit up to one extent or another. Generally speaking it's nothing to worry about, especially if the baby is thriving and gaining weight. He'll most probably grow out of it by the time he's twelve months old.

If your baby is one who spits up, try burping him a bit more frequently during feedings to expel any air he may have gulped along with his milk. Feed him in a relatively upright position, and keep him sitting up for twenty or thirty minutes after he's finished. Raise the head of his crib to keep his body elevated when he's lying down. You might also check to make sure that the holes in the nipples on your baby's bottles are neither too small nor too large. Intense crying before feedings or too much jostling during a feeding can contribute to spitting up. Before you get upset about your baby spitting up, think about his eating patterns. Do any of them contribute to his spitting up? If so, try to modify them. Of course, if his spitting up remains a concern, talk to your doctor.

Is it GERD?

Gastroesophageal reflux disease (GERD) is an uncomfortable, often painful condition that develops when the muscle that closes off the stomach isn't working as it should. Food that goes into the stomach comes back up along with stomach acids, causing heartburn. Unlike the healthy, happy, growing baby who spits up, a baby with GERD is likely to be irritable; he might suddenly begin crying or cry constantly. He'll arch his back; he might refuse to eat or he might choke or gag when he eats; or he might cry in pain when he spits up. He's a baby in pain. And he may not be gaining weight as he should. If you suspect that your child is in pain because of GERD, speak with your doctor.

What causes it?

Vomiting is fairly common in small children. It is often related to overeating, overexertion, or anxiety. Vomiting can also be caused by acute gastroenteritis brought on by the rotavirus, a virus affecting the digestive tract (page XX [X-Ref]). Food-borne bacteria in tainted food can be a source of vomiting; it is basically the body's way of ridding itself of something it should not have. Vomiting can be triggered by the sight or smell of decayed food, motion sickness, or seeing another person vomit. It's not uncommon for a child to vomit after a strong coughing fit. Bouts of vomiting don't generally last very long. They are often more uncomfortable and unpleasant than dangerous.

Vomiting may be a symptom associated with an underlying disease. If so, your child will experience other symptoms along with vomiting. Pain in the lower right side of his lower belly along with vomiting may indicate appendicitis; vomiting along with a stiff neck may be related to meningitis. If your child has a headache along with dizziness and vomiting following a fall or head trauma, it may mean he has a concussion. It's important to speak to your physician or health care provider if you believe that his vomiting is associated with any of these conditions.

How You Can Help

There are several ways to help your child manage his discomfort. The first is to calmly reassure him that he'll be alright. Help your child rinse out his mouth with clear water to help him get rid of the sour taste that often follows vomiting.

While you may not be able to stop him from vomiting, you can help to prevent dehydration. Give your little one very small amounts of an oral rehydration fluid, such as Pedialyte, to keep him hydrated. You can offer a baby 1 to 3 teaspoons of fluid every 10 minutes using a teaspoon or an oral syringe. If he is able to hold down the fluids, slowly increase the amounts to 2 to 3 tablespoons several times an hour. But don't give him more rehydration fluid than he'd ordinarily eat at a feeding. If he only takes 3 ounces at a feeding every 2 hours, don't give him more than 3 ounces of Pedialyte over a 2-hour period of time. Once he can hold down clear fluid feed him as you normally would. Start to give him smaller amounts of his normal intake to make sure that he's able to hold it down.

Try giving your older baby or child up to 1 ounce of clear fluids every 15 minutes until it's clear he can keep down the fluids. Offer him diluted juice or a frozen diluted juice pop in addition to the oral rehydration fluid.

Once your child can keep fluids down you can offer him easily digestible, bland foods such as bananas, rice, cereal or crackers, applesauce, or toast. Milk products and foods that are high in fat and sugars are difficult to digest, so try to eliminate them until his belly feels considerably better.

If you find that your child overeats at a single meal, try giving him smaller meals more frequently throughout the day.

If motion sickness sets him off, don't allow him to eat a full meal before getting into a car or bus.

Watch him. What do you think sets off his bouts of vomiting? Think about it; modify his behavior—or yours—and speak to your doctor if necessary. You may have more power over his digestion than you may think.

Treatment

This treatment can be used for the child who is vomiting, spitting up, or has GERD. In each of these cases, your child's energy is moving up toward the face and head. This treatment is aimed at bringing the energy back down to where it belongs—into the stomach and lower belly. You want to calm the digestive system and you want to calm the child. By massaging the chest, abdomen, and back in a downward direction, you are working to bring the energy to the lower reaches of the digestive tract.

All of the shaded areas in the treatment illustrations are useful in helping your child to feel better. Some areas are shaded lightly, others somewhat darker. The lightly shaded areas need the least amount of work; the darkest areas need the most attention. Work on the lightly shaded areas just once or twice during the course of the treatment; work on the darker areas more frequently, staying at each area no more than 3 to 5 seconds at a time. When you treat an older child, adolescent, or adult, you can locate the acupoints within the darkly shaded areas. But when you treat a baby or young child, working generally in the area of an acupoint will produce the desired result.

Use a gentle touch when you massage your child. When you are working on a baby, all the pressure that's needed is the degree of pressure you would use if you were finger painting or checking to see if a cake is finished baking. If your child is sick and vomiting, wait until after he's calmed down and cleaned up before treating him.

Take your time; make him comfortable; relax.

1. Start with a gentle massage of your child's chest and stomach. Massage in little circles directly on the breastbone and down over the belly. Start at the chest and end a bit below the belly button.

   Conception Vessel 10, 11, 12, 13, and 14, lying between the navel and the sternum, are all used to help relieve stomach fullness and vomiting.

2. Gently massage the outside of the lower leg from the knee to the ankle. Give a bit more attention to the area a couple of inches below the knee.

   The Stomach meridian lies on the outside of the lower leg. Stomach 36 tones all aspects of digestion and elimination and helps to strengthen the system in general.

3. Massage the inside of the foot from the arch to the base of the big toe.

   Spleen 3 and Spleen 4 are used to treat digestive upset and pain.

4. Massage down the middle of the front of the arm starting at the elbow and working down toward the center of the palm.

   Pericardium 3, 5, 6, 7, and 8 are used to treat digestive upset, pain, and vomiting.

5. Massage the muscles each side of the spine that lie on the lower part of the ribcage beginning next to the bottom of the shoulder blade and moving toward the lower back.

   Bladder 17, 20, 21, and 22 are used to treat indigestion and vomiting.

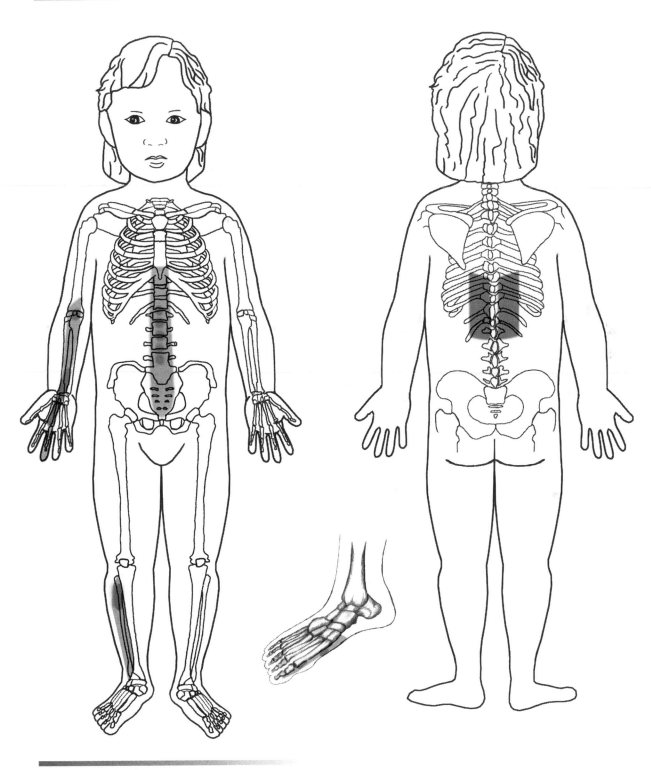

Treatment areas on the front,
back, and foot for vomiting

Irritability, Fussiness, and the Inability to Sleep

When should you check with your doctor?

If your child is irritable and fussy and looks or acts sick or injured, call your doctor. If all of your efforts at soothing your child are unsuccessful and she is crying inconsolably for an hour or more, check with your doctor. If your child is crying on and off for a day or more for no apparent reason, check with your doctor. If your older child's inability to sleep interferes with her daily activities, talk with your doctor.

And it's important to take care of yourself, too.

If you begin to feel frustrated and unable to control yourself in the face of a fussy, irritable, crying baby, know that you're not alone. Every parent has gone through the frustration of not being able to soothe a crying baby. Take a break if you can. Hand your baby off to somebody else—if there's no one else around, put her in her crib, check to make sure she's safe, and leave her alone for a while. She may just cry herself to sleep.

What Is It?

Your children experience their stresses and strains not very differently than we adults do. Infants and babies communicate their discomfort by crying and being fussy. The toddler may be whiney and have tantrums. The older child may act out if she's under stress or is fearful. Some may be able to communicate their fears or stresses but may not be able to manage them on their own.

What Causes It?

It is not uncommon for a baby or young child to go through a fussy period when she is beginning to come down with an illness or when she is uncomfortable because she's hungry or has a stomachache, if she's teething, if she's too hot, too cold, or too tired. And sometimes young children are just stressed. With infants and small babies, an environment in which there is a lot of activity and stimulation can lead to irritability and fussiness. The endless visual and auditory stimulation of a brightly lit room with a large screen television or the ongoing activity of older siblings can be a bit much for a baby. So can being around large groups of people; parties can be stressful events for small children—even their own birthday parties.

With older children, family dynamics, relationships with their brothers and sisters, the demands placed upon them by their teachers and their schoolwork, and issues with friends can be stressful, and it can be difficult for them to express or manage by themselves.

Children of all ages are intuitive. If mom and dad are feeling stressed, their children will feel it and will likely fear it. This can be a common source of a mild underlying fear that may be the source of irritability and the inability to sleep.

How you can help . . .

. . . make her more comfortable

Check your baby for the usual things that might be making her physically uncomfortable: a wet or soiled diaper, hunger, uncomfortable clothing or body temperature, or being overtired.

If your baby is going through a period of fussiness or irritability, try to keep activity down to a minimum when she's in the room. Keep the television off. When you are feeding her, interact with her quietly. Play some quiet music. Sit with your baby in a dimly lit room. Cuddle her, rock her, read to her, talk to her in soothing tones.

You know your child better than anyone else. If your older child seems stressed or frightened about something, talk with her. Ask her if she knows what's bothering her and see if she'll talk with you about it. Sometimes just talking about a problem is the best solution. If you can remember how you felt when you were her age, you will understand how she feels. Talking with her binds the two of you together. It reminds her that you are there to help her and be there with her. Often just knowing that is calming in and of itself.

. . . prevent problems from snowballing

Keep a close eye on your baby or young child. Her fussiness might be the first sign that she's getting sick. Look out for early signs of infection or disease that may warrant seeing your doctor. Nipping something in the bud often speeds the healing process.

Create a place in your home that is the "quiet place" for your infant or young baby. It might be a chair where you sit together in a corner of a room, or a place in her room. You can turn it into the place that she feels the most calm and the most at ease. Take her there at the first signs of distress or irritability. Sit with her or quietly read to her. If you get into the habit of going to the same quiet place, she'll get into the habit of calming herself when she's there.

Help your older kids to unwind and let go of the stresses of their day. This will take different forms for different kids. Some kids need to run around and burn out pent-up energy after a day at school; some kids might just want to relax around the house for a while to wind down. Figure out what your kids need and help them work it through.

Try to avoid over-scheduling your kids after school. Somehow, these days it seems that there is hardly any time for a kid to just be a kid. Between music lessons, karate, computer classes, tutors, dance lessons, and homework, so many children seem to be as stressed as the most type-A financial wizard on Wall Street.

Avoid stressful conversations during dinner. Eat, talk, relax—digestion will be better for everyone.

Allow your kids to rest as much as they can; help them to relax before they go to sleep so they sleep well through the night and awaken refreshed. Encourage them to avoid computer games or activities, homework, stressful family conversations, and violent television or video games before bed. Just as you need to clear your head and wind down before bed, so do our kids.

Develop a bedtime routine. The familiarity of routine can be very calming to a child. If you get your children into the habit of whatever bedtime routine you are comfortable with, that in and of itself will help them to wind down. For some children a warm bath an hour or so before bed, followed by reading and quiet talking, sets the stage for a good sleep.

Most kids need in the vicinity of ten hours of sleep a night. Encourage your kids to go to bed early enough to get their ten hours so they can wake up refreshed and clear headed. Having a regular bedtime can avoid the "I don't want to go to bed" fights that disrupt many families so many nights a week. If your child is not ready for sleep, let her stay awake and read quietly in bed until she gets sleepy—but make sure she knows that she's to stay in bed.

A word on diet

Some kids become keyed up when they've eaten too many products made with refined white flour and sugars. In general, try to limit your child's consumption of sugary foods and drinks, specifically in the evening hours.

If you are breastfeeding, try to avoid drinking green and black teas, coffee, and colas, and avoid eating chocolate. All of these contain caffeine. Children can be very sensitive to the effects of caffeine—their bodies are small. If your child tends to be irritable or have difficulty sleeping, consider the possibility that she is taking in caffeine, possibly from a variety of unrelated sources. Perhaps that is a contributing factor. Look into her diet and modify it if you need to. There are many caffeinated beverages available to children—colas, sports drinks, energy drinks, chocolate drinks, flavored green and black teas and iced teas, ice tea mixes, and caffeinated water. Even Mountain Dew, 7-Up, and Sunkist orange soda contain caffeine. Coffee flavored ice creams and frozen yogurts also contain caffeine. Chocolate contains sugar as well as caffeine and can really keep your kids going.

As a guideline, consider limiting your older child's caffeine consumption to 50 milligrams daily—approximately the amount in 12 ounces of cola.

Treatment

Use this treatment whenever you see that your baby or child is getting irritable. You don't have to make it a formal treatment time, and it doesn't have to take longer than a couple of minutes. A gentle stroke here and there throughout the course of a fussy day may take the edge off for both of you. A soothing stroke of the chest and back or a gentle massage of the head and neck might be enough to calm your child and ease her discomfort. You can cradle your baby in one arm and use the other to massage her feet or her hands while you're gently rocking her in your favorite glider or rocking chair. Slow, gentle strokes are all you need. If your older child is having trouble falling asleep, by all means do the treatment just before bed. The soft strokes will help to calm you both.

The shaded areas in the treatment illustrations show where to work on your child to help calm and soothe her. Some areas are shaded lightly, others somewhat darker. The lightly shaded areas need the least amount of work; the darkest areas need the most attention. Work on the lightly shaded areas just once or twice during the course of the treatment; work on the darker areas more frequently, staying at each area no more than 3 to 5 seconds at a time. When you treat an older child, adolescent, or adult, you can locate the acupoints within the darkly shaded areas. But when you treat a baby or young child, working generally in the area of an acupoint will produce the desired result.

Use a gentle touch when you massage your child. When you are working on a baby, all the pressure that's needed is the degree of pressure you would use if you were finger painting or checking to see if a cake is finished baking.

Take your time; relax.

1. Begin by gently stroking your child's upper chest, beginning at the top of the breastbone and moving down toward the upper stomach.

   Emotional energy is held in the upper chest. Massage of the area releases this energy and softens the pectoral muscles, which will help calm the breathing.

2. Lightly press the point on the breastbone that lies midway between the nipples. Lightly press the point just beneath the break in the ribcage.

   Conception Vessel 17 is used help open the chest. Conception Vessel 14 is used to calm.

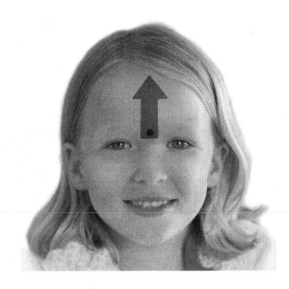

Treatment areas of the face for irritability

3. Gently stroke the forehead, beginning between the eyebrows and moving up toward the hairline.

4. Lightly press the point between the eyebrows.

   Extra point Yintang is used here to calm the system.

5. Beginning at the temple, lightly massage in an arc around the ear, ending at the bottom of the skull.

   A gentle massage of the head and scalp is one of the most relaxing experiences a person can have. Gall Bladder meridian, which traverses head many times, is said to hold emotional energy. Perhaps it is the release of that energy that explains the relaxing effects of a scalp massage (or a good shampoo at the hairdresser!). Gall Bladder 20 at the base of the skull is used to calm.

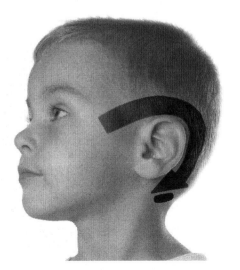

Treatment area of the head for irritability

6. Massage the inside of the forearm beginning at the elbow and working down toward the little finger. Focus your massage just above the wrist, down through the pinky side of the palm, and on to the little finger.

   Heart meridian is used to calm the mind. Heart 6 and Heart 7, located just above the wrist fold, are used to treat irritability and insomnia. Heart 7 is used with Pericardium 6 and Spleen 6 to calm and soothe.

7. Massage the inside of the forearm above the wrist fold, in the center of the wrist.

   Pericardium 6 is used with Heart 7 and Spleen 6 to calm and soothe.

8 Massage the back side of the hand in the web between the thumb and index finger.

   Colon 4 is used with Liver 3 to calm the system.

9. Massage the inside of the lower leg a couple of inches above the inside anklebone.

   Spleen 6 is used with Heart 7 and Pericardium 6 to calm and soothe the mind.

10. Massage the top of the foot, focusing the massage between the long bones that attach the toes to the foot. Focus on the space between the big toe and the second toe.

    Liver 3 is used with Colon 4 to calm the system.

11. Gently stoke down the back of the neck and across the shoulders.

    Release of the trapezius muscle will release much of the tension that is held in the upper body. Each of the yang meridians travels through this area. Release of this area contributes to the free flow of energy through the system.

12. Stroke down the back, in the musculature beside the spine. Focus your massage at the area between and just below the shoulder blades.

    Release of the erector spinae muscles will have the added effect of calming the chest and upper stomach as well as the back. It will help to open and release the breathing.

13. Massage the lower back just above the pelvis.

    Massage here will help to bring energy down from the upper body into the lower body and belly, soothing and calming your child.

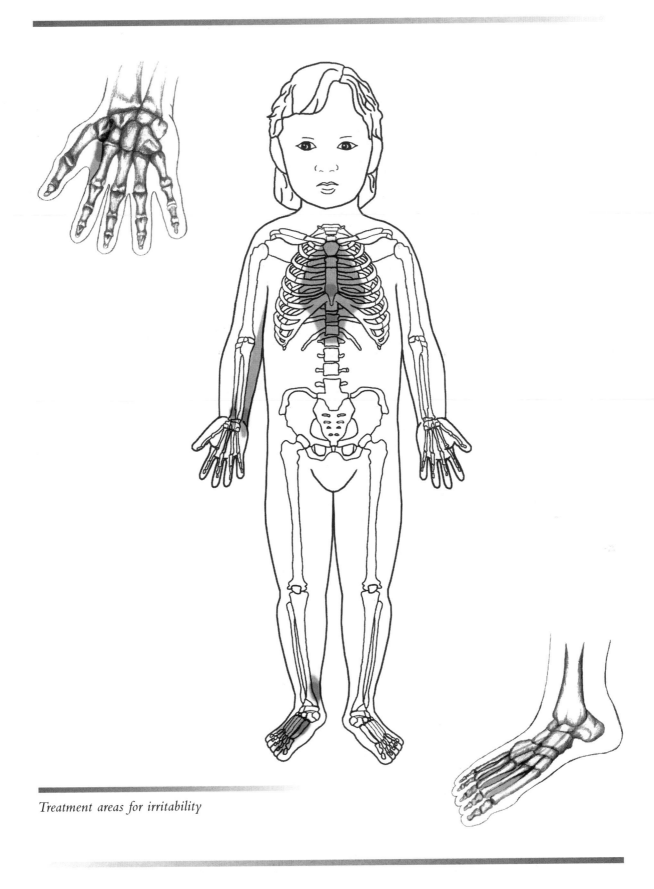

Treatment areas for irritability

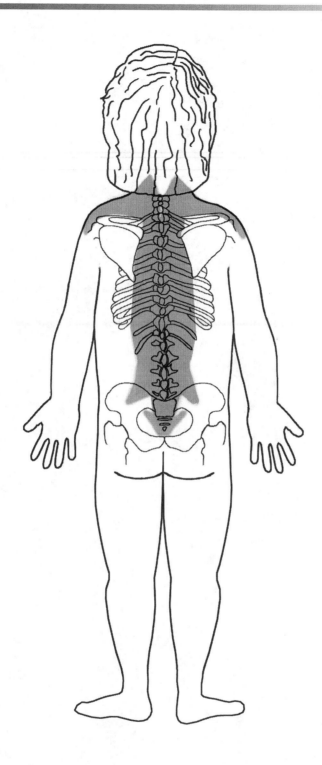

Treatment areas of the back for irritability

Colic: Excessive Crying

When should you check with a doctor?

If you think your baby's crying is the result of an injury, or if your baby has blood or mucus in his stools or has very hard stools, consult with your doctor.

We all need help sometimes

Infancy can be a very difficult period in *your* life. If you believe that *you* have reached the end of the limit of your patience listening to your baby cry, regardless of whether or not you believe the crying is due to colic, speak to your doctor or other health care provider. Coping mechanisms, support groups, and other forms of help can be obtained to get you through what may be a very difficult period.

What is it?

Every newborn infant cries. It is the infant's way of communicating his need to be fed, burped, comforted, and cleaned in this utterly new world in which he has found himself. Crying is normal for babies, particularly for babies between birth and three months of age.

For some of them the crying is at its worst in the late afternoon, early evening, and nighttime hours. Perhaps it is because by that time of day the infant's developing nervous system has been overloaded with stimuli. Remember that *everything* the baby sees, hears, feels, touches, and senses is completely new for him. That's a lot of stimuli in any one day.

Many infants cry inconsolably for several hours a day, often for apparently no reason that has been determined. These babies are healthy, well fed, and well cared for, and yet beginning at around 3 weeks of age they begin a pattern of crying that is very distressing for a new parent to live through. The crying resists all attempts to be calmed by the very loving, well-meaning but exhausted and frustrated new parents. This is a baby who is experiencing colic. Whether you want to believe it or not, colic is considered to be the extreme end of normal crying behavior.

A baby who has colic will cry at the same time of day, usually in the late afternoon, evening, or nighttime hours. The loud, often piercing cry starts and ends abruptly and usually lasts for two to four hours several days a week, for several weeks at a time. A colicky baby is colloquially defined by the rule of 3's—the baby who cries for three hours a day, three days a week, for three weeks in a row is considered to be a colicky baby. He might pull his knees up and tense his fists; his belly may get really tight and hard, and he may appear as if he's in pain. Calming him may seem impossible. He may pass gas or have a bowel movement toward the end of the crying period. Fortunately, for everyone's sake, this pattern of crying peaks at about six weeks and usually ends by the time he is three or four months old—with no harm done to your beautiful baby. It's your frayed nerves that will take the greatest brunt of the trauma during this colicky period.

What causes it?

No one really knows what causes colic. What is known is that it is not caused by anything the parent is or is not doing; colic isn't your fault. It has nothing to with whether or not you are breastfeeding your baby. The gas the baby expels when he's in a colicky period has led to the thought that colic is related to an immature digestive tract, but the reality of that hasn't been demonstrated. Babies take in air when they cry—the gas may be just that. Numerous possibilities have been studied—none has been shown to be the cause of colic. Colic just happens to some babies.

How you can help . . .

. . . yourself

The single most important thing you can do to help your baby is to help yourself, to nurture yourself. In many cases, your baby is just a few weeks old—you've just given birth. And regardless of whether you've had a vaginal birth or the abdominal surgery known as a Cesarean section, YOU need to heal. You may be exhausted, overwhelmed and in pain. Understand, first, that you are not a superwoman and you cannot and *should not* take care of everything. The best way to take care of yourself is to get help if you need help with other aspects of your life—your work, school, or older kids.

Know, too, that you, as a parent, are not the cause of your baby's crying. Parents of colicky babies often become frustrated, angry, depressed, disappointed. This was not what they were expecting when they thought about bringing their new little bundle home. And yet colic is normal for so many of these little bundles. They will grow out of it. This will pass. Take one day at a time. Sometimes you need to take one hour at a time, knowing always that that hour will pass. If you find yourself becoming depressed, angry, or tending toward violence, seek out help and support from your partner, your caregiver, your community, and your family and your friends. If all you need is a few hours away from the baby, take the time. Remember, you can't help your baby if you aren't healthy and as relaxed as possible yourself.

. . . your baby

I'm a firm believer in being close to your infant, carrying him, holding him, touching him. Thinking about what your baby is experiencing from his point of view explains why. Your infant was inside your body for the entire time he was developing; you essentially grew a body part. Then birth occurs, and your baby is no longer a part of your body. Nothing is familiar to your baby any more. Where is the constant pulsing? Where is the warmth? Where are the whooshing sounds he heard? We bring him home from the hospital and he's placed in a bassinet or crib. He is somehow expected to be comfortable for hours at a time in this new large, cold, unfamiliar place, separate from everything that he was a part of.

I believe that physical contact with your new baby is crucial for him and crucial for you. Hold him often for the first couple of months, respond quickly to his cries, carry him, let him feel your body as he gets accustomed to this new world. Will this prevent your baby from experiencing colic? Perhaps. Perhaps not. But it seems to me that it will make your baby more comfortable and peaceful as he gets used to being a separate entity. You can't spoil an infant. You can let them know that you are there for them and will always be there for them, doing your best to soothe and comfort them.

Keep your baby in a quiet, peaceful environment. Sometimes babies react to a noisy, hectic atmosphere in which there is a lot of activity and people coming and going. Just like a lot of other human beings, your child may be one who needs peace rather than activity.

Try a variety of soothing techniques used through the ages. Try swaddling—some babies find comfort in the tightly wrapped blankets, holding their arms tight beside the body. Try compressing his belly—whether you are holding him tightly against your body chest to chest, placing him belly down across your lap, or holding him like a football—belly down across your forearm—compression against belly can be a great relief to some babies. It may also help the baby to pass gas. Rhythmically pat his low and mid back. Patting the back, alone or while compressing the belly, gives some babies a bit of relief.

Swaying while holding your baby in your arms can be soothing to your baby. Rocking your baby is comforting—sometimes to both of you. If you get tired there are a variety of infant swings that can replace your arms for minutes at a time. Taking your baby for a car ride or a walk around the block can help. Sounds such as white noise or the drone of a vacuum cleaner or washing machine can help. The sounds of soothing music—fine, soft classical guitar, a favorite of mine—has also been known to work.

Soothing a crying baby is a process of trial and error. You have to figure out what your baby likes and what he doesn't like. It requires patience, and in some cases nerves of steel. But rest assured, this period will give way to another sooner or later. This is likely to be the first of many trials that you will have to go through as a parent. Our parents did it with us. Now we know what they went through, and can appreciate them just that much more.

Treatment

All of the shaded areas in the treatment illustrations are useful in helping your child to feel better. Some areas are shaded lightly, others somewhat darker. The lightly shaded areas need the least amount of work; the darkest areas need the most attention. Work on the lightly shaded areas just once or twice during the course of the treatment; work on the darker areas more frequently, staying at each area no more than 3 to 5 seconds at a time. Remember that when you massage your infant the gentlest touch is all that's needed.

We want to accomplish two things with this treatment. The first is to calm your baby and the second is to calm your baby's digestive tract. Given that, the best time to treat your baby is not when he is in the midst of an episode of colicky crying. Treat him when he is more relaxed. You can work on him when you are feeding him or simply holding him. When he is in the midst of a crying jag and you are walking around with him, rocking him or holding him tightly against your chest to compress her abdomen, massage the areas of the back, feet, and legs that are shaded in the following illustrations.

Try and keep yourself calm and massage him gently. Your emotional state will come through your hands. He'll feel your desire to help. Be patient. And be compassionate—for both of you.

1. Start by gently stroking your baby's forehead from the midpoint of the eyebrows up toward the hairline.

2. Press very lightly on the point that lies between the eyebrows.

   Extra point Yintang is used here to calm the system.

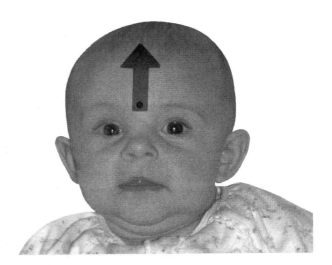

Treatment area for colic

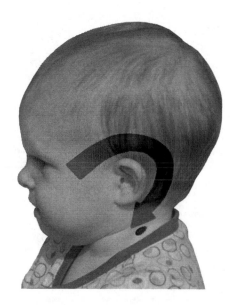

Treatment areas of the head
for colic

3. Stroke around the ears starting at the temples and working around to the back of the head.

    A gentle massage of the head and scalp is one of the most relaxing experiences in the world. Gall Bladder meridian, which traverses the head many times, is said to hold emotional energy. Perhaps it is the release of that energy that explains the relaxing effects of a scalp massage (or a good shampoo at the hairdresser!). Gall Bladder 20 at the base of the skull is used to calm.

4. Gently massage the midline of the body from the breastbone down through the stomach and into the abdomen. Do this several times, using slow, gentle movements.

    Stroking the midline will bring energy out of the upper torso and into the lower body.

5. Gently massage the upper stomach, beginning just underneath the breastbone and ending just below the belly button.

    Conception Vessel 14, below the breastbone, is used to calm the system. Conception Vessel 12 helps to regulate the digestion.

6. Massage the muscle on both sides of the belly button, working toward the lower belly. You might find that there are tiny areas of tight muscle in that region.

    Trigger points in the rectus abdominis muscle have been identified as a possible source of digestive upset and colic in infants.

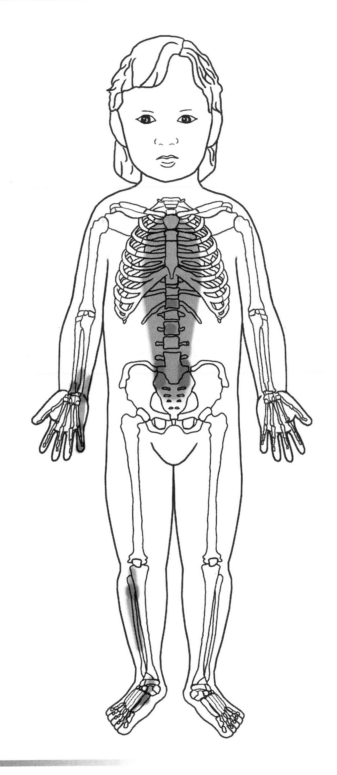

Treatment areas for colic

7. With the baby's hand turned palm up, massage the pinky and the pinky side of the palm of the hand and the side of the upper wrist.

   Portions of the Heart meridian lie on this part of the hand. Heart 7, Heart 8, and Heart 9 help to calm.

8. With the baby's hand turned palm up, massage the area 1 inch or so above the wrist fold in the center of the arm.

   Pericardium 6 works with Conception Vessel 12 to regulate digestion.

9. With the baby's hand turned palm down, massage the area 1 inch or so above the wrist fold in the center of the lower arm.

   Triple Heater 5 acts to calm digestion.

10. Gently massage the web between the thumb and the index finger.

    Colon 4 works with Stomach 36 to balance digestion.

11. Massage a couple of inches below the knee on the outside of the lower leg.

    Stomach 36 works with Colon 4 to balance digestion.

12. Gently massage the space between the long bones connecting the first and second toes to the foot.

    Liver 3 works with Colon 4 to calm the system.

13. Gently massage between the second and third toes and the long bones that connect the toes to the foot.

    Stomach 44 helps the descending action of digestion.

14. Gently massage the baby's back in a downward direction on both sides of the spine, from just below the shoulder blades to the sacrum, the flat bone at the bottom of the spine.

    The downward massage of the Bladder meridian will help to calm the baby. A bit of extra attention to the area just above the pelvis, Bladder 25, will stimulate the colon helping the baby to pass gas if need be.

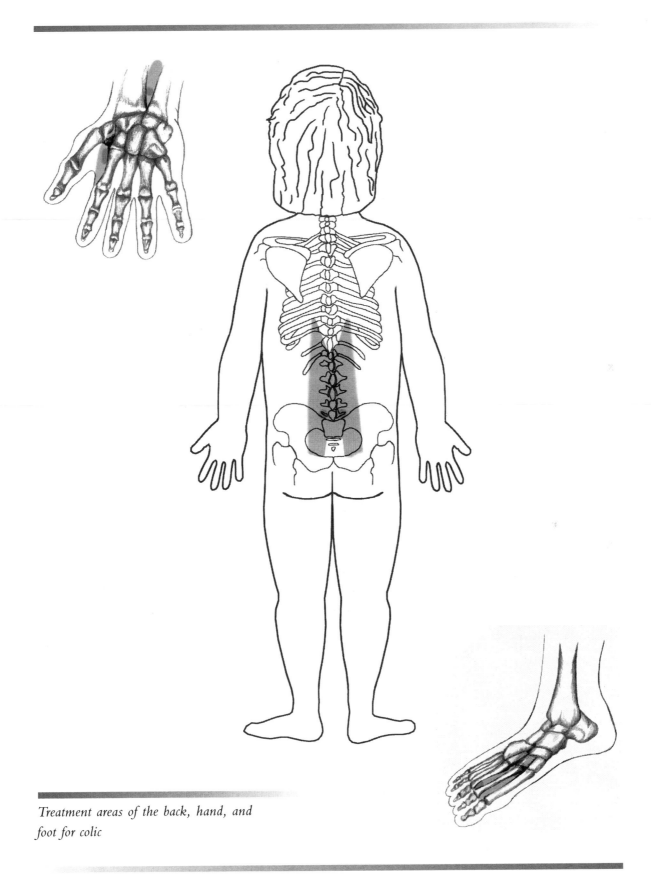

Treatment areas of the back, hand, and
foot for colic

Urinary Tract Infection

When Should You Check with Your Doctor?

If your infant has a fever without any apparent cause or in combination with vomiting and/or diarrhea and persistent irritability, or if your older child develops fever and chills in combination with abdominal and low back pain call your doctor.

If you suspect that your child has a urinary tract infection, check with your doctor.

What is it?

A urinary tract infection is an infection of one or more organs of the urinary tract. The urinary tract produces urine, the body's liquid waste. The urinary tract consists of the *kidneys,* the two bean-shaped organs that filter the blood and extract waste; the *bladder,* the balloon-like organ that holds urine until it is passed from the body; the *ureters,* the long tubes that connect the kidneys to the bladder; and the *urethra,* the tube that leads to the outside of the body and through which urine passes.

The most common urinary tract infection is *cystitis,* an infection of the bladder. A bladder infection is an inflammation and infection of the lower part of the tract. When bacteria enter the urethra they may migrate up to the bladder, which may lead to an infection. Bladder infections are easy to eliminate with the use of antibiotics. But if the infection goes untreated, the bacteria may migrate to the kidneys and cause a kidney infection. A kidney infection is far more serious than a bladder infection. An untreated kidney infection can lead to permanent kidney damage or kidney failure, particularly in infants and children under two. It's important to see a physician if you believe that your child has a urinary tract infection.

Babies, toddlers, and older children may show varying symptoms when they have a bladder infection. Infants and babies may simply have a fever. They might be irritable and fussy. They might vomit. They might have diarrhea. They may just seem sick. Toddlers and older children are likely to have some of the more typical symptoms of bladder infection: odd-smelling urine or cloudy or bloody urine. They may urinate in small amounts much more frequently than normally. They may tell you that it hurts when they have to urinate, or they may cry when they urinate. Little ones may have "accidents" even when you were sure that their toilet training days were over. If a kidney infection develops, your child may have many of the same symptoms of a bladder infection but she might tell you that she also has pain in the belly and back or has pain on the side below the ribs. She might have fever and chills and she might look and act very sick. That child needs to see a doctor right away.

What causes it?

Bladder infections are much more common in females than in males, because in females the rectum, the urethra, and the vagina are so close to one another. In females, the urethra is short and placed near the opening of the vagina; in males it is longer and ends at the end of the penis. Urine normally does not contain bacteria. However, the digestive tract is filled with bacteria. Some promote proper digestion. Some, like *Escherichia coli* bacteria (E. coli), live in the intestines, where they serve to maintain a healthy colon. These are the bacteria that are found in feces. These bacteria find their way onto the skin near the urethra when the area is not sufficiently cleaned after a bowel movement. When they migrate up the urethra and into the bladder they can cause a bladder infection.

Bubble baths or using strong soaps can irritate the urethra. That irritation can lead to an infection.

Sometimes there is a physical abnormality in the urinary tract that causes recurrent urinary tract infections. If your child has repeated urinary tract infections, your doctor will want to perform diagnostic tests to determine the source of the infections.

How you can help . . .

. . . make her comfortable

Offer her plenty to drink. Water is ideal for flushing the system. Cranberry juice helps tremendously to keep the bladder flushed. A substance in the cranberry prevents bacteria from adhering to the wall of the bladder. Most commercial cranberry juices have very high sugar contents, so try diluting the cranberry juice with purified water or look for naturally sweetened brands that aren't as sweet.

If your little girl is having trouble urinating, encourage her to take a warm bath. The warm water is soothing to the genital area and it will help her pass urine more easily.

Reassure her that this will pass. She may want to avoid urinating because of the discomfort it causes. Encourage her to drink a lot and pee a lot because urinating will help to cleanse the bladder and help make the infection pass quickly.

. . . prevent it

When your baby soils her diaper, clean her carefully and thoroughly from front to back. Check all those little nooks and crannies around those pudgy little legs to make sure that she's completely clean.

Encourage your kids to go to the bathroom as soon as they feel the need to urinate. Little kids play and play until the very last minute. This is not the best thing for the bladder. Urinating is one way that bacteria are flushed from the system.

Teach your little girl to clean herself carefully from front to back after using the toilet. Use unscented white toilet tissue. Toilet tissue with scents and dyes can be an irritant to sensitive areas.

Teach your kids to wash and dry their genital areas thoroughly when they bathe. Discourage bubble baths and the use of harsh soaps or soaps with chemical scents or dyes.

Dress your little girl in cotton underwear. Encourage her to promptly change out of wet clothing, such as bathing suits and leotards. Women of all ages should learn that a warm, dark, moist place becomes a friendly home to unwanted organisms that won't make you happy in the long run.

If your child's urine is frequently dark yellow, encourage her to drink more purified water throughout the day. The urine that we pass should be relatively colorless at least once daily. Urine that is regularly very dark is highly concentrated urine, which can be an irritant to the bladder. It can also be a sign of mild dehydration.

A word on diet

Offer her cranberry juice daily. It doesn't have to be much. A few ounces of cranberry juice, diluted with purified water can be a helpful preventative.

If your child is eating solid foods, encourage her to eat fruits and vegetables. The fluid and fiber content in fruits and vegetables will help her digestive tract and her urinary tract to function well.

Treatment

This treatment can be used to help your child feel more comfortable while she is recovering from her infection. It will help the body heal itself quickly.

All of the shaded areas in the treatment illustrations are useful in helping your child to feel better. Some areas are shaded lightly, others somewhat darker. The lightly shaded areas need the least amount of work; the darkest areas need the most attention. Work on the lightly shaded areas just once or twice during the course of the treatment; work on the darker areas more frequently, staying at each area no more than 3 to 5 seconds at a time. When you treat an older child, adolescent, or adult, you can locate the acupoints within the darkly shaded areas. But when you treat a baby or young child, working generally in the area of an acupoint will produce the desired result.

Use a gentle touch when you massage your child. When you are working on a baby, all the pressure that's needed is the degree of pressure you would use if you were finger painting or checking to see if a cake is finished baking.

Work on your child any time she's open to it. Take your time; relax.

1. Begin with a gentle massage of the chest and abdomen, starting at the center of the chest and working down to the lower belly.

    Massage of this area will serve to relax the abdominal musculature in the mid and lower body.

2. Gently massage the lower belly. Massage in a downward direction, beginning on either side of the belly button and massaging down toward the legs.

    Massage here will soften and release the lower abdominal musculature. Trigger points in the abdominals may develop in the presence of a bladder infection.

3. Gently press the point that lies between the break in the ribcage and the belly button.

    Conception Vessel 12 helps to open the midsection of the body.

4. Gently press the point that lies slightly below the belly button.

    Conception Vessel 6 helps to regulate the lower warmer.

5. Gently massage the area above the pubic bone.

    Conception Vessel 3, 1 inch or so above the pubic bone, is used in the treatment of genitourinary disorders. Conception Vessel 4, 1 inch above Conception Vessel 3, is used in the treatment of genitourinary disorders.

6. Massage the back side of the hand between the index finger and the thumb.

    Colon 4 works with Kidney 7 to help strengthen immune function.

7. Massage the inner thighs, starting at the top of the inner thigh and working down to the area just below the knee. If you can manage to massage this area you'll be in good shape—it's likely to tickle your little one silly. If you keep your palm flat on her inner thigh as you massage her, you'll have a better chance of succeeding.

    Massage here will encompass the area of the Liver and Spleen meridians. The areas on the inner thigh, both above and just below the knee, Spleen 10 and 11 and Liver 8 and 9 are used to treat bladder dysfunction.

8. Massage the outside of the lower leg just beneath the knee.

    Stomach 36 works with Spleen 6 to strengthen immune function.

9. Massage the inside of the lower leg a couple of inches above the inside anklebone.

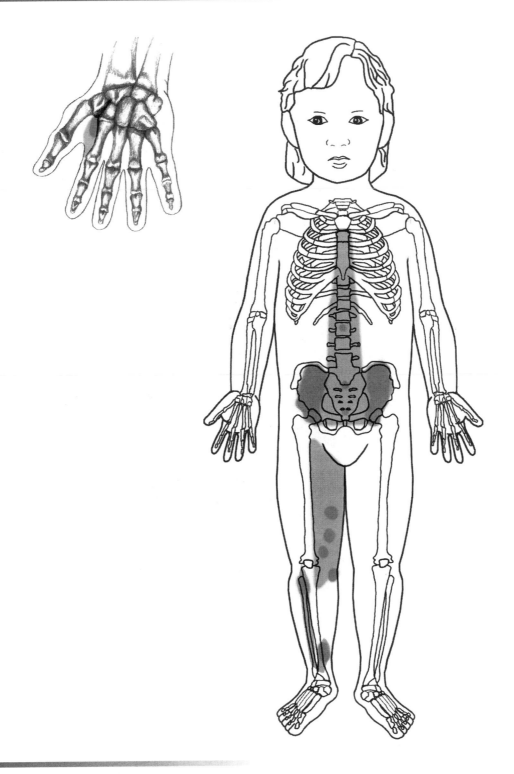

Treatment areas for urinary tract infection

Spleen 6 works with Stomach 36 to strengthen immune function. Spleen 6 works with Conception Vessel 3 to balance bladder function.

10. Massage around the outside of the ankle and down the outside edge of the foot toward the toes.

    This area will encompass points that control the functioning of the bladder. Bladder 63 and Bladder 64 at the base of the fifth metatarsal directly affect the bladder and are used in the treatment of bladder dysfunction.

11. Massage around the inside anklebone.

    Kidney meridian points lie close to the inner anklebone. Treatment here will support kidney function. Kidney 7 works with Colon 4 to help support immune function.

12. Massage the small of the back from the bottom of the ribs to the top of the pelvis.

    Massage here will encompass Bladder 52, which will help to strengthen kidney function.

13. Massage the sacrum and right over the little dimple where the sacrum connects to the pelvis.

    Bladder 28 is traditionally used with Bladder 58 to treat bladder infections.

14. Massage the backs of the thighs beginning at the bottom of the buttocks and working down toward the back of the knees.

    Good luck. This is another very ticklish area. If you succeed you will help to support bladder function.

15. Massage the outer part of the back of the knee fold.

    Bladder 39 promotes the movement of fluids throughout the urinary tract.

16. Massage the outer part of the bulky calf muscle just where it meets the thin Achilles tendon.

    Bladder 58 is traditionally used with Bladder 28 to treat bladder infections.

17. Complete your treatment with a gentle stroking of the back.

    It feels good and will relax both you and your little one.

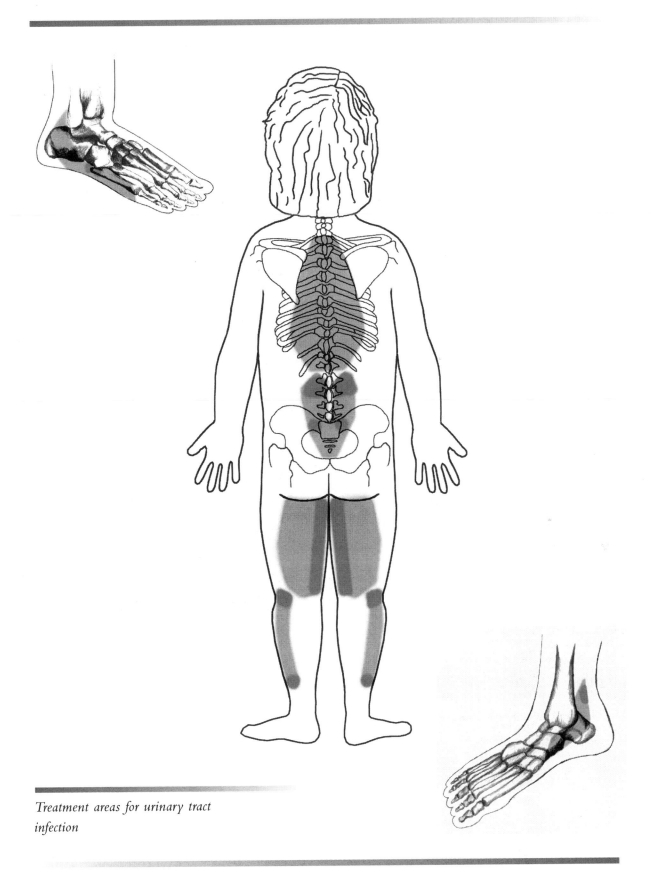

Treatment areas for urinary tract infection

Aches, Pains, Bruises, Sprains, and More

When should you check with your doctor?

If your child has injured himself and is unable to move, stand, or support his weight, or if he has joint or bone deformity, seek medical attention as soon as possible.

If he has swelling or bruising that continues to increase after twenty-four hours, or if he has a swelling or lump in a muscle that does not cause pain and persists for more than seven days, consult your physician.

If you have any question as to the severity of an injury, it is always best to check with your doctor.

Our muscles, tendons, ligaments, and bones, along with the tissues that connect and support them, allow us movement. Every movement we are physically capable of, large and small, simple and complex, is because of the ingenious placement of our muscles on our bones. When muscles are healthy they are supple, elastic, soft, and pliable; their contraction and release take place easily and painlessly.

When muscles contract, they move the bones that they connect to. In fact, we would be completely incapable of movement without muscles. That includes the movement that takes place when we are breathing, digesting, and eliminating; when our blood is being pumped through our arteries and veins; when the pupils of our eyes are opening and closing, and any other movement you can think of.

Movement is natural. Just look at your child. On a good day, when he's feeling well, all he wants to do is move. Most of the time children move without having any pain at all, but periodically an injury might occur that causes some discomfort. Injuries range in severity from the mild muscular soreness after hauling around a heavy backpack to the intensity of a fractured or broken bone.

Those two types of injuries require very different kinds of attention and treatment. A fracture requires medical treatment, while most often a muscle strain or a bruise does not. And then there are the rest of the injuries that fall in between those two.

What is common to all types of muscle and skeletal injuries is that it is not only the injured area that is affected—the various muscles and joints that work along with the injured area are affected as well. A simple pulled muscle will have an affect on all the muscles in the region; a far more serious fracture will do the same thing.

We can't change the injury. But we can help the muscles to heal by using massage, moist heat, ice and rest.

Let's take a look at some of these types of injuries.

Listen to your body

The body's aches and pains tell us something. For example, when we injure a foot, it hurts. The pain is the body's way of telling us not to walk on that injured foot too much. When we mask the pain through the use of an over-the-counter analgesic or an anti-inflammatory, we open ourselves up to exacerbating an injury because we do things that we wouldn't and couldn't do if we were aware of the pain.

When your child sustains an injury, use non-steroidal anti-inflammatories (NSAIDS) cautiously. Mild discomfort may not warrant their use. They may reduce the pain and inflammation in the first hours of an injury, but NSAIDS may also increase the total amount of time the body requires for complete healing.

Bruises. Everybody experiences the occasional bruise. A bruise, known as a *contusion,* is caused when tiny blood vessels in the soft tissue under the skin are broken. As most of us well know, you usually get a bruise from a fall or bump or getting hit with an object. The blood within those vessels seeps into the surrounding tissue and causes a "black and blue" mark under the skin. Usually it starts off as a red or purple bump that turns blue or black after a couple of days. As the body heals itself the bruise turns from blue to yellow to brown, and then it disappears completely.

Most minor bruising doesn't require any special healing measures. But you can help reduce bruising and inflammation after an injury through the use of ice pack placed on the area for 10 to 15 minutes soon after the injury occurs.

Muscle spasms. A *spasm,* or *cramp,* is a sudden and involuntary contraction of a muscle that causes a painful, hard, bulging in the muscle. Your child may awaken from sleep with a painful calf or foot cramp. Muscle spasms or cramps are usually caused by muscle fatigue or imbalances of calcium, magnesium, or potassium. They are not uncommon in children.

Cramps and spasms are usually temporary and can be relieved with slow stretching, the application of moist heat or ice, and gentle massage to the area. Walking often helps to release a foot or calf cramp. If your child tends to have cramps, try to make sure that his diet includes an ample variety of fresh fruits, vegetables, whole grains, dairy, and protein, as well as sufficient water. If he sweats a great deal, he might also benefit from an electrolyte replacement drink after strenuous exercise.

What are growing pains?

Your child complains of an aching in his legs that comes and goes. It may last for days. Why is that?

Has he had a bit of a growth spurt recently? If he has, he may be experiencing growing pains. The long bones of the legs grow more quickly than the muscles that attach to them. His muscles are straining to catch up. These are growing pains.

Gently massage his legs; add a bit more protein to your child's diet; increase his fluids, and encourage some rest. They should pass within a week or so.

Strain. A *strain* is an injury to the muscles or to the tendons, which attach muscle to bone. A strain is often caused by overusing the muscle. It's fairly atypical for a very young child to have this kind of muscle injury. Their muscles are supple, elastic, and fluid. But if your school-age child has just begun to carry a heavy backpack to and from school or if your older child or teen is an athlete enthusiastically practicing a sport, he might experience a muscle strain.

When a muscle is strained, there will be pain in the area when your child moves—but if he doesn't move the area he won't feel any pain. His muscles may feel tight in surrounding areas, and he may have some swelling over the area of the strain.

There are mild, moderate, and severe muscle strains.

A mild strain is known as a pulled muscle. Most of the time a pulled muscle will heal itself in a few days. You can help your child with the discomfort of a mild muscular strain by encouraging him to soak in a bath of warm water with or without Epsom salts. Using a moist heating pad on the area for 20 minutes at a time once or twice a day also helps the healing of a mild strain.

A moderate strain is referred to as a torn muscle. Some of the muscle's fibers or portions of the tendon attaching the muscle to the bone are torn. If your child has a torn muscle, he won't have the same strength in that area that he had prior to the injury. It takes a couple of weeks, at a minimum, for a torn muscle to heal completely.

A severe strain is the rupture of the muscle-tendon-bone attachment. That level of injury requires surgical repair and about six to ten weeks' healing time.

If your child has a moderate or severe muscle strain, use R.I.C.E.—rest, ice, compression, and elevation—as first aid within the first twenty-four hours after his injury. If you believe your child has torn a muscle, see your doctor for evaluation.

Even the most mild strain can lead to taut, hardened, tender bands and trigger points in the muscle. What we think of as "knots" in the muscle are trigger points. It's important to work on the muscle to help the strain heal, and then once it has healed, eliminate the taut bands and trigger points in the muscle. Gentle massage to the strained muscle and the area it affects will help its healing tremendously. It will help to increase circulation to the area and reduce areas of tightness in the vicinity of the injured muscle. Movement will become easier and less painful, and the muscles will return to their normal elastic, supple state.

When should I use heat?

As a basic rule of thumb, if a muscle is pulled or mildly strained or if your child is simply sore from overusing his muscles, use *moist heat* rather than ice. The application of a moist heating pad, one that produces moisture against the skin, is very soothing to sore muscles. It's important to avoid using dry heat, such as a heating pad—dry heat dehydrates the muscle and delays recovery. Soaking in a bath of warm (not hot) water is very soothing to sore muscles, and the addition of Epsom salts is great for the muscles.

Tendinitis. *Tendinitis* is an inflammation of a tendon, the structure that attaches muscle to bone. Tendinitis may develop in your older child from overusing the muscle through repetitive use (doing the same action over and over again), or taking part in a sport without stretching and warming up. How common is that for our teenaged athletes and dancers?

An inflamed tendon will be swollen, painful, and tender. The region will generally ache. Pain is worse with movement and may be worse at night. There may be heat and redness over the tendon where it attaches to the bone.

Common sites for tendinitis are the elbow, shoulder, knee, and ankle. Our young tennis players may develop "tennis elbow," tendinitis at the elbow; our pitchers may develop tendinitis at the rotator cuff, more commonly known as tendinitis of the shoulder; our basketball players may develop "jumper's knee," tendinitis at the knee; our runners and dancers may develop Achilles tendinitis, tendinitis of the Achilles tendon at the back of the heel.

R.I.C.E. is the best formula for self-care of tendinitis: rest, ice, compression, and elevation. Stress the rest part of this formula.

Massage of the muscle connected to the tendon will help the tendon by releasing the force of the muscle pulling against it. Bringing blood to the area through the use of massage will speed healing time.

What is R.I.C.E.?

R.I.C.E. is a term that describes first aid for an injury. It is an acronym for the terms REST, ICE, COMPRESSION, and ELEVATION. Used within the first twenty-four hours after an injury, the R.I.C.E. formula will help to reduce inflammation, and the heat, redness, swelling and pain that accompanies it.

REST means that you need to stop using the injured part. Rest it.

ICE is the application of ice to the injured area. Ice can be applied in many forms: in a plastic bag covered with a soft towel; a bag of frozen peas that will conform to the contours of your body; a reusable gel pack. Whichever form you use, you should cover it with a soft, dry towel to prevent the skin from getting wet. Keep ice on the area for 10 minutes; remove it for 20 minutes. Repeat this cycle three times—so one period of icing will be 90 minutes long. Ice can be applied 2 or 3 times a day within the first twenty-four to forty-eight hours after an injury. It is extremely useful in the treatment of joint injuries and tendinitis.

COMPRESSION is the placement of a light pressure bandage on the area to help to keep swelling to a minimum. An elastic bandage can be used to lightly wrap the injured area. You have to be careful when you wrap the injury—the wrapping shouldn't be so tight that it increases the pain or cuts off circulation.

ELEVATION indicates the need to raise the injured part above the level of the heart. This helps prevent swelling.

Ice should be used within the first twenty-four hours to help the healing of a bruised muscle or an injured tendon, ligament, or joint. Ice helps to reduce swelling and inflammation.

Sprains. A *sprain* is the overstretching of one or more ligaments within a joint. Ligaments attach bone to bone; they are important because they are part of the support structure of the joint itself.

If your child has a sprain he might describe feeling a popping or tearing at the joint. The joint will be very tender, swollen, and bruised. He will be in a lot of pain.

There are mild, moderate, and severe sprains.

With a mild sprain, some of the fibers of the ligaments are torn. There isn't any loss of the function of the joint, but healing time may still be between two and six weeks.

A moderate sprain involves a rupture, or tear, of a part of the ligament. The ankle joint may be unstable and need immobilizing in order to heal. Healing time may be as long as six to eight weeks.

A severe sprain is the complete rupture or separation of the ligament from its attachment on the bone. Surgical repair is required for a severe sprain, followed by complete immobilization of the joint. Healing time may be as long as two to six months. Because ligaments have an extremely limited blood supply, healing time may take as long as it would take to heal a fracture, and sometimes even longer.

The ankle and the knee are common sites for torn ligaments. An older child who is an athlete or a dancer might develop a sprain at some time in their youth. If they do it is extremely important to allow adequate time for rest and healing before returning to their activity. This might be quite a challenge for some avid young athletes! That being said, encouraging your child to rest and heal will avert the possibility of future joint instability and repeated, increasingly severe, sprains.

If you believe that your child has suffered a sprain, have him evaluated by your doctor. Immediate first aid for a sprain is the application of R.I.C.E.—rest, ice, compression, and elevation—particularly within the first twenty-four hours. Once the doctor has determined the extent of the sprain, you can help your child heal from his sprain by massaging the muscles connecting to the joint. For example, if he's sprained his ankle, massage his legs, concentrating on the muscles of his lower legs and feet.

Dislocation. When the bones that form a joint separate from one another, a *dislocation* has occurred. Some dislocations are momentary and correct themselves on their own; some require medical intervention to be repaired. If your child has suffered a dislocated joint that did not self-correct, there will be an obvious visible deformity of the joint and he probably won't be able to use the joint. In other words, if he's dislocated his knee, it won't look like a knee should look and he won't be able to move or bend it. There will be tenderness, swelling, bruising and possibly numbness.

Immediate first aid is the use of R.I.C.E., particularly within the first twenty-four hours. If you believe that your child has dislocated a joint, have your physician evaluate him as soon as possible. Muscles surrounding a dislocated joint are frequently strained to one degree or another. Once the immediate local pain and inflammation of the dislocation has been reduced and joint healing has begun, massage will help to increase circulation and release the muscles that have been affected in the area. Working on the muscles will help them to regain their normal strength and to prevent future muscle weakness in the area.

Fractures. A crack or break in a bone is a *fracture*. If your child fractures a bone it is likely that he will have sudden and extreme pain, swelling, and tenderness in the injured area. There is usually a change in appearance of the injured part: blood under the skin and possibly a protruding bone. The broken bone—the arm, leg, or finger—may be bent out of shape. A fracture can occur to any bone. Some fractures require surgical intervention in order to stabilize the bone; others require splinting or casting in order to maintain the proper position of the bones until healing begins.

It is necessary to obtain medical care as quickly as possible in the event of a fracture. Most fractures require a cast to prevent movement of the body part and allow the bone to knit properly. Once the cast is removed, massage will help those muscles regain their previous strength.

Treatment

While this likely needs to go unsaid, if you suspect that your child has sustained any serious injury, have him evaluated by a physician before treating him with massage. If you are treating him for discomfort that is not alleviated within forty-eight hours, have him evaluated by a physician.

Massage helps your child heal from an injury that he sustains. Muscles involved in the injury will often develop taut, stringy bands and trigger points, or knots, within those bands. The muscle will become tight, and it won't contract or stretch as it should. Once that happens, a domino effect occurs. Put simply, when one muscle can't do its job, the muscles it works with to move an area have to work harder or differently. The improper functioning of those muscles then affects the workings of some other group of muscles. This frequently leads to chronic pain or dysfunction in an area that may be so subtle at first that it goes unnoticed, sometimes for years.

Young children bounce back quickly because their muscles are so supple and soft. But as they get older the shadows of past injuries become more pronounced. Working on an injured muscle and the muscles that are affected by it is one way to deter the dominoes from falling.

When you massage your child's sore muscles, use a gentle touch, but one that is strong enough to feel the muscles give way under your fingers when you compress them. Use your fingers to feel the difference between soft areas of the muscle, areas that feel swollen or warm, and areas of the muscle that are tight and feel like bands or hard knots. Those are taut bands and trigger points. It's best to avoid massage over a swollen or warm area, but you can gently compress tight muscle bands and knots with your fingertips when you encounter them. Compressing tight muscles may feel somewhat tender to your child, but the muscle will soften if you press it gently enough to feel its resistance under your hand. You can hold the pressure for a slow count of 5 to 10. Don't press too hard or too long if your child is experiencing pain from the work you are doing. What you don't want to do is pass your finger back and forth over a taut band as if you were plucking a guitar string. That never really releases the muscle. All it does is hurt.

Treatment of the Neck

Make sure to see your doctor if your child has neck soreness or pain that does not change in three to five days. If your child has neck stiffness and pain and a fever of 102°F or more, see your physician.

There are many ways that the muscles in your child's neck may become sore and painful. Your child might complain of neck pain if he is overworking the muscles by carrying a heavy backpack, if he's fallen asleep with his head and neck in a weird position, if he spends hours in front of a computer, or if he's stressed. A whiplash-type injury will affect the muscles of the neck; whiplash occurs often in unexpected situations like car accidents or falls, and even from those impacts that are expected—like those that take place during football practice. Certain activities, including bicycling, wrestling, and weight lifting, can be tough on the neck. And a child who has asthma or any recurrent respiratory problem that makes it difficult to breathe may have neck tightness and soreness.

When a person has restricted neck muscles with trigger points, it is not uncommon to experience headache, facial pain, facial pressure, and jaw pain in addition to neck tightness and soreness. Work on your child's muscles if he has any of these symptoms. If they are relieved after you've massaged his neck and upper back, you can be fairly certain that the pain came from those tight muscles.

It's easiest to massage your child's neck when he's sitting with his

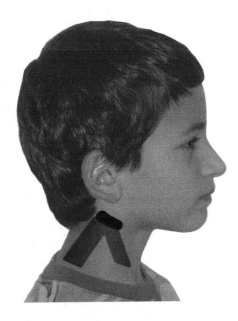

Massage and trigger points for the treatment of neck pain

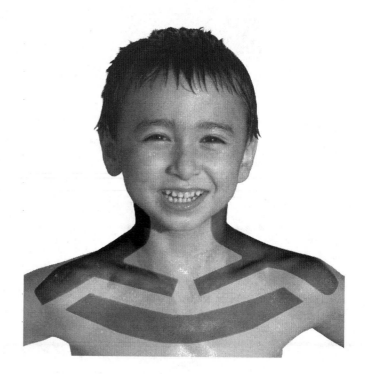

Massage and trigger points of the upper body for the treatment of neck pain

back facing you. Work on both sides of his neck and back. You'll be able to compare the two sides, making it easier for you to hone in on the taut, tender bands of muscle tissue that are the source of his problem.

A massage of the neck will include the muscles of the back of the neck, the sides of the neck, the base of the skull, the upper shoulders, upper back, mid back, and upper chest.

Massage will affect the release of restrictions and trigger points in the upper, middle and lower trapezius, levator scapulae, cervical and thoracic paraspinal muscles, the scalenes and sternocleidomastoid muscles.

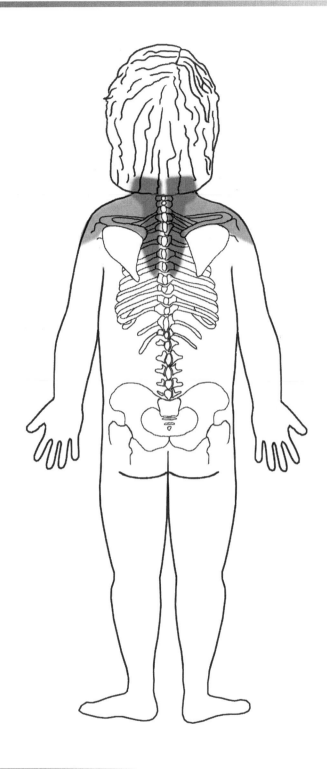

Massage and trigger points for the
treatment of neck pain

Treatment of the Shoulder

If your child has shoulder soreness or pain that does not change in three to five days, check with your doctor to make sure that his pain is muscular. If your child's had a serious injury, if he is in a great deal of pain, if there is sudden swelling and bruising, or his shoulder looks deformed, seek medical evaluation.

Athletics is probably the most common source of shoulder and upper arm pain in children and teens. Overuse of the muscles in the shoulder is not uncommon for avid tennis players, basketball players, swimmers, and baseball players (especially pitchers). Weightlifters and wrestlers may overwork the shoulder and arm muscles as well. Anyone can injure the shoulder muscles by trying to break a fall, by walking a dog that is pulling against a leash, and by hauling around a monstrous backpack.

The shoulder is amazingly complex. Muscles that work on the shoulder attach to parts of the back and to parts of the front of the body. You'll have to work on both sides when you work on your child. You can work on your child while he is sitting down or while he is lying down.

If your child has shoulder and /or upper arm pain, you'll be working on his upper shoulders, his upper back, shoulder blades, the muscles between his shoulder blades, and the spine, the lower back, his upper chest, and upper arm. Look for taut bands on his upper shoulders, both on and on top of the shoulder blade, and in the deltoid, the muscle that caps the shoulder, giving the shoulder its characteristic shape.

Massage will affect the release of trigger points and areas of restriction in the upper trapezius; three of the rotator cuff muscles (supraspinatus, infraspinatus, and teres minor); latissimus dorsi; teres major; pectoralis major; pectoralis minor; anterior, middle, and posterior deltoid; biceps brachii; and triceps brachii.

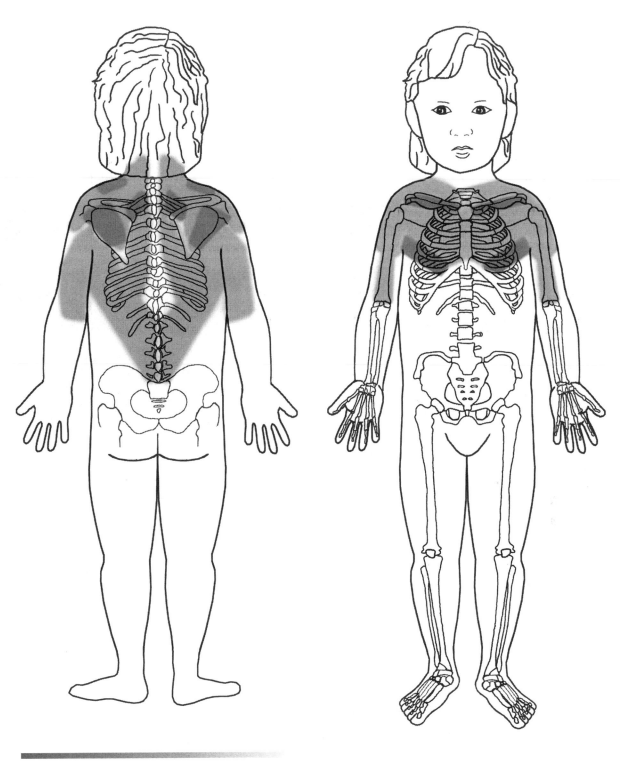

Massage and trigger points for the treatment of shoulder pain

Treatment of the Elbow and Wrist

If your child experiences an acute injury with intense pain, bleeding, or severe bruising, visible elbow joint deformity, numbness of the fingers, inability to use the elbow, hand, or fingers without pain or loss of circulation to the hand and fingers resulting in their discoloration, consult a physician for medical evaluation.

Children under four years of age sometimes develop what's called "nurse-maid's elbow." The well-meaning adult may pull the child's straightened arm, causing a slight dislocation of the bones of the elbow. If your very young child seems to be experiencing elbow pain or the unwillingness to bend or use the arm, see your physician.

Elbow and wrist pain due to muscular tightness is often related to grip. This is true of both children and adults. The young tennis player may be gripping the racquet too tightly, or the handle of the racquet may be too wide for his small hands. Another source may be related to the intensity with which your little one is gripping his pencil or pen when he's writing—particularly in the early phases of learning how to write. Believe it or not, overuse of video games can do the same thing. In each case the force of the grip tightens the muscles of the forearm. Trigger points, or knots, can develop in those muscles, and elbow pain can result.

When you massage your child's arm, both you and he will be most comfortable if you are sitting down facing one another. Massage his left arm with your right hand and his right arm with your left hand.

Start at the outside of his arm just below the elbow. Try to use your thumb to make small circles, starting with the muscles above the elbow and working down toward the wrist. Work on the front of the forearm as well as the back of the forearm. Try to feel the difference between the many long bands of muscle that lie along the length of the forearm. Some will seem quite tight compared to the others. When you locate a tight area in the muscle, press gently for a slow count of 5 to 8 to release the muscle. There may be areas of tightness in many of the muscles throughout the forearm.

Massage of the forearm is aimed at the release of restrictions in brachioradialis and the extensors and flexors of the hand and fingers.

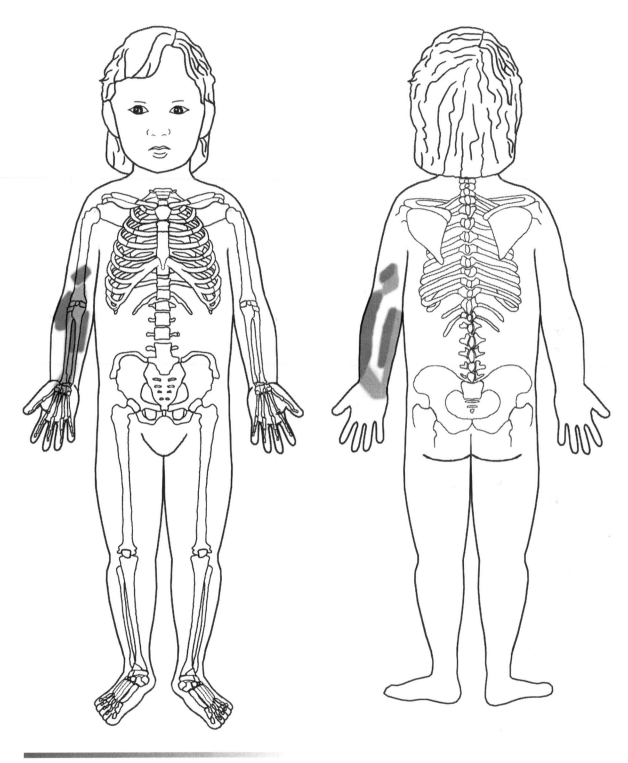

Massage and trigger points for the treatment of elbow and wrist pain

Treatment of the lower back

See your physician as soon as possible if your child has sustained an acute injury or if his pain is due to trauma; if his pain is severe or constant; if he is unable to bear weight due to pain; or if pain is accompanied by numbness, tingling, or loss of strength in the legs and feet or loss of bowel or bladder control.

If his moderate pain is accompanied by fever and chills or is not alleviated within three or four days, have him evaluated by a physician.

Lower back pain is happily fairly uncommon in our children. Most at risk are our dancers, gymnasts, martial artists, football players, and wrestlers. As generally supple as our children are, much to their credit, the amount of work and effort that they apply when they are engaged in their physical art will sometimes cause their muscles to become strained and sore. The overuse and overstretching of the muscles of the back, hips, and buttocks can lead to pain that is felt in the lower back. Extremely tight hamstrings can also lead to lower back pain. Some of our teenaged boys are ready to work out but reluctant to stretch. When the hamstring muscles are very tight they can pull on the lower back. Check out the hamstrings to see how tight they are when you are working on your child. If he needs to, make sure he stretches the hamstring muscles on the backs of his thighs and the muscles on his inner thighs, the adductors.

When you massage your child you will work on his middle and lower back in the muscles that lie just beside the spine, and on his buttocks, his hips, and the hamstring muscles on the backs of his thighs. Feel for areas of tightness within the muscles; both tight bands of muscle and muscle "knots" can be compressed to help them to release. When you compress an area of tightness in a muscle, hold the pressure for a good count of 10 to 15. The larger muscles in the buttocks, hips, and thighs will require a bit more pressure than the smaller, thinner muscles that lie on the upper body.

Trigger points and taut bands in erector spinae, quadratus lumborum, gluteus maximus, gluteus medius, gluteus minimus, piriformis, and the three hamstring muscles (the biceps femoris, semitendinosis, and semimembranosis) can cause pain and restricted range of motion in the lower back and hips and sometimes in the thigh and leg.

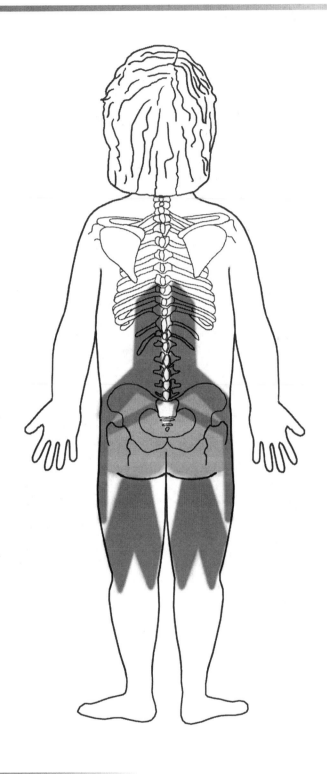

Massage and trigger points for the treatment of lower back pain

Treatment of the Thigh and Knee

If your child has had a serious injury or trauma, if there is swelling, bruising, heat, or redness at the knee, or if he is unable to bear his weight, seek medical evaluation. If your child has knee soreness or pain that does not change in three to four days, have it evaluated by your physician.

Knee pain is not uncommon in late childhood and adolescence. It can stem from many sources, one of which is overuse and strain of the muscles of the thigh and leg. Some of the largest, longest, and strongest muscles in the body act on the knee joint, and these are the very same muscles that are involved in the heavy work of athletics— running, jumping, and kicking. Add to that the fact that the knees, along with the ankles, carry the weight of the entire body, and you can understand how hard the knee works.

If your child has knee pain you will want to massage the muscles that connect his hips to his knees and his knees to his lower legs. You'll need to work on both the front and the back of his leg. Start with your child lying on his back.

Massage the outside of his thigh from the hip to the knee. Look for areas of tightness and tenderness from the middle of the outside of his thigh to just a couple of inches above his knee. When you find an area of tightness, compress it for a good count of 5 to 8. Repeat the same process with the inner part of his thigh, looking for areas of tightness just a couple of inches above the inner knee Massage right along the top of his thigh from the hip to the knee. You might find areas of tightness closer to the hip than the knee in this part of the muscle.

Once your child turns onto his belly, you'll massage the back of his thigh and the upper part of his calf, looking for areas of muscle tightness and tenderness.

All of the areas described may be the source of pain in the knee. They are also areas that tend toward tightening following an injury that affects the knee. Whether your child has knee pain or stiffness, or if he's recovering from a knee injury, working on these muscles will be beneficial to him.

Massage of the thigh will release taut bands in the quadriceps group: vastus lateralis, vastus medialis, rectus femoris; the adductor group: adductor magnus, adductor longus and brevis; the hamstring group: biceps femoris, semitendinosis, and semimembranosis; and gastrocnemius.

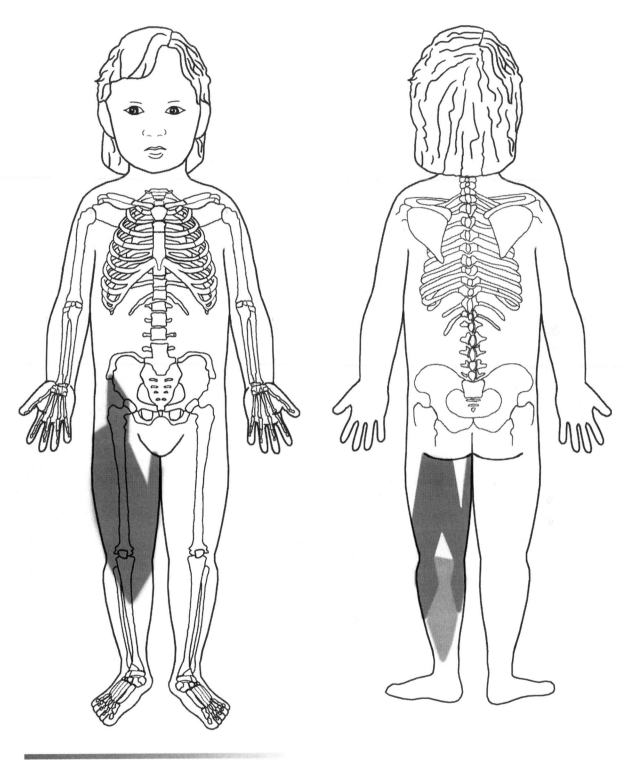

Massage and trigger points for the treatment of knee pain

Treatment of the Ankle

If your child has had a serious injury or trauma, if there is swelling, bruising, heat, or redness at the ankle, or if he is unable to bear his weight, seek medical evaluation. If your child has ankle pain that does not change in three to four days, have it evaluated by your physician.

Ankle injuries are probably one of the most common injuries sustained by children and young athletes. Whether jumping off a curb or on a trampoline, bicycling, using a scooter or skates, or dancing around the house, it's fairly easy to roll onto the outside of the foot, causing an ankle injury. The injury may be as simple as a strained muscle or as complex as an ankle sprain or fracture. Whatever the case, you can help your child's ankle pain by caring for the muscles that support and move the ankle.

Begin to work on your child's ankle while he is lying down on his back. Place a pillow under his knees so you can easily reach all the muscles of his lower leg. The many muscles that you will work on help to support and stabilize the ankle joint. Start on the outside of his lower leg just below his knee. Massage in between the large bone of his lower leg: the tibia and the smaller, thinner fibula lying on the outer part of the leg. Begin under the knee and work down toward the outside of the ankle. Look for areas of tightness in the part of the muscle close to the knee and then a few inches above the outside anklebone. Gently massage around the outside anklebone, using a very light and gentle circular motion.

Massage *up* the inside of the lower leg, massaging at the curve just below the inside of the knee.

Work on the back of the lower leg when you've finished working on the front. Work through the thick upper part of the calf, looking for areas of tightness in the outer and inner part of the calf muscle. Massage down toward the lower part of the leg, where the muscle becomes thin and connected to the Achilles tendon. When you get closer to the ankle, look for areas of tightness in the muscle beside the Achilles tendon, just above the ankle.

Massage will affect the release of tibialis anterior; peroneus longus, brevis, and tertius; gastrocnemius; and soleus.

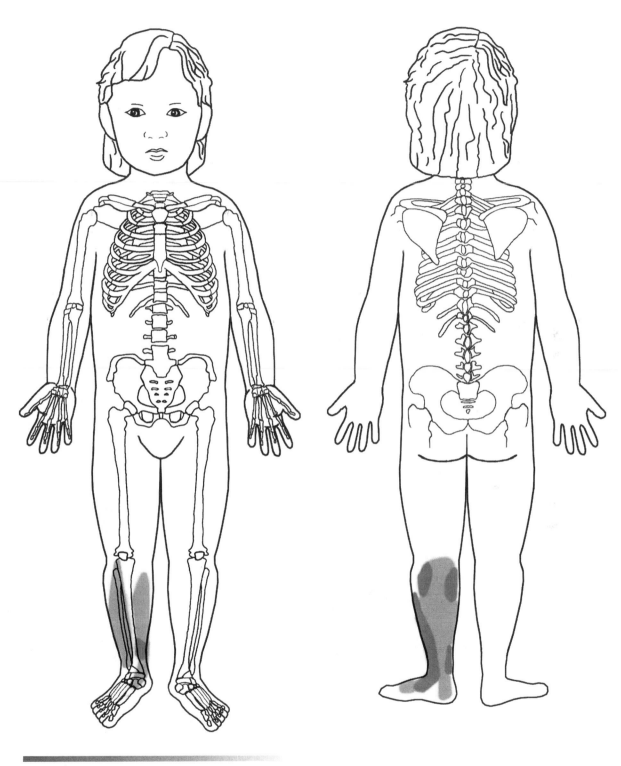

Massage and trigger points for the
treatment of ankle pain

Epilogue

The Ever-Flowing Fountain
and the Four Cardinal Needs

When we talk about health, we often think only about the physical aspect of health: physical fitness, strength, vitality, the proper functioning of the organs, the absence of disease. But far more goes into being healthy than taking care of the body. A human being is a complex interplay of the body, the mind, and the emotions. Emotional and mental well-being must be cultivated, along with physical fitness, in order to attain a state of real health.

Your child, your precious gift, requires so much of you. As parents we give to our children, hoping that our influence will help them grow into clear-thinking, emotionally balanced, physically healthy, responsible adults. When you're trying to conceive, and while you are in the "I want to have a baby" stage, it's not uncommon to have given little thought to the fact that not only will you have a baby (who will place enormous demands on you), but that baby will become a child (who will place enormous demands on you), and then an adolescent (who will place even more enormous demands on you), a teenager (who will place even greater demands on you), a young adult (phew! almost there!), and one day, an adult with a family of his or her own.

A parent is like a fountain that is continually giving forth, continually flowing. Like a fountain you are giving of yourself, providing for your children. It begins when you've given a bit of your body to create this new life: a sperm and an egg. A piece of dad and mom have made this baby. It then continues when the baby is developing inside the mother's body. Your body is providing nutrients, blood, fluids, and a warm environment in which to develop and grow. Once the baby is born you are still providing. But in addition to food and nutrients, you are providing what I believe are the four cardinal needs: care, love, support and guidance.

Becoming a parent is exhilarating, joyful, and sobering. In giving birth to another human being, you implicitly take a vow to care for, love, support, and guide the human being that is brought forth into this world by virtue of your desire. As strong as marriage vows are, these vows are just that much stronger. They are writ in your blood and tissue. A child *needs* care, love, support, and guidance. While he may survive without it, he cannot *flourish* without it.

As your baby grows, she keeps changing. And as she changes her needs change. As a parent, like the fountain you keep providing, giving forth, but what you give and how you are giving it must change as surely as your baby changes. The parent of an infant must be different than the parent of a two year old; the parent of an eight year old must be different than the parent of a two year old; the parent of a teenager has to be different than the parent of a child, on and on throughout the course of your child's life until the moment when you realize that your child is an adult and she doesn't need a parent anymore—at least not in the ways that you've focused on up to this point. And yet, as your child reaches adulthood, it's likely that you'll find that your desire to remain connected, to give, almost never stops. It just changes over time.

Raising a child is like cultivating a garden. Through every changing season, and at various points within each season, your garden needs something different from you. Impatiens can't be planted in late fall, and it makes no sense to harvest your tomatoes before they've ripened in late summer. Every gardener knows that you must act in sync with the changing needs of your garden. You aren't leading that dance, the garden is; Mother Nature is. Just so, in raising a child you must be willing to yield, to defer, to your child's changing needs. You must be willing to keep in step with him as his attitudes evolve and change, all the while keeping your aim in mind: to care for, love, support, and guide. As a parent your children need to know that you are there for them, to care for them (whether they think they need it or not), to love them (whether they think they want it or not), to support them (whether they think they want it or not), and to guide them (whether they think they need it or not).

Your ongoing efforts to love, care, support and guide will not ensure success, but it will help to create a path that may make it possible for you to move in sync together throughout the course of your lives.

Care

We all know what basic care of an infant involves: you clothe the baby to keep her warm, feed her to help her body grow, shelter her by giving her a place to live; you keep your baby dry and warm, changing his diaper when he is wet or soiled, feeding him when he is hungry. If you are reading this book, you already know that these are the essentials. Now think about this: in order to *truly care* for your child, you need to *look* at him and *see* him in order to *understand* what he needs. You see, caring for your child's emotional well-being is as necessary as caring for his physical well-being.

Whenever you get the chance to think of it, whether in a moment of hurt or sickness, frustration or joy, put yourself in your child's place. Ask yourself how you would feel if you were in his little shoes at that moment. Consider, if you were him, what you would want. Once you've thought that through, let that determine how you act toward him.

To do this in earnest you must first, and quite intentionally, put aside *your* desires in that very same moment; you have to put aside *your* needs and wants and focus on your little one. You might need or want to help or soothe him in a particular way, but he may not be responsive to it just then. When you are really caring for your child, you let go of your needs and meet his.

If you carried in your heart and acted from the Golden Rule, "Do unto another as you would have another do unto you," parenting would be so much easier, for parent and child alike. But parenting from within this tenet is both incredibly simple and awfully difficult at the same time. It's difficult because it requires *being present* for your child when you're with her. As strange as it sounds, in order to place your child's needs above your own, you have to actively remember that you are the adult, the parent, and that she is the child. Isn't that what parents are supposed to do? Many of us have seen a three year old standing next to his mother calling "Mommy! Mommy! Mommy! " as she talks on the phone to a friend. She yells at the child: "Can't you see I'm on the phone?!" You might think to yourself: Why doesn't she just ask her friend to hold on a minute and ask the child what he needs? At that moment you recognize that the child is a child, and that he needs to be given attention at that moment, before his frustration leads to a melt down. It would only take a moment.

But how many of us are guilty of doing just exactly the same thing? Maybe you are in the middle of making dinner, or watching television, or working on the computer or just coming home from work and want absolutely nothing else but to change clothes and settle down to shake off the stress of the day. We do it without thinking; we aren't sufficiently present within ourselves to remember that we are the parents and he is the child. It requires a mental effort to be present for your child.

Try very hard to be aware of what you are feeling when you are dealing with your child. If you can see that you might be feeling frustration from your day at work *before* you are faced with taking care of baby, you might be able to set those frustrations aside rather than taking them out on your child. If you can see that you are really angry about a conversation you just had with someone, maybe you won't yell at your child for some minor event. Taking care of your child really begins with knowing what is going on inside of *you*. If your mind is lost in thinking about work or something else that you imagine you should be doing, you can't present for him. You can't be there to really care for your child.

Take a moment to think about your childhood. Do you carry something in your memory that was said to you or that you experienced that stayed etched in your heart and mind? Children are amazingly impressionable; the smallest thing can stay for a lifetime. These are unintended injuries, emotional scars left by something a parent or teacher says in an offhand way: "You are so silly"; "Don't be stupid"; "You never shut up! "; "You're a real sourpuss"; "Leave me alone already! " Or things that were said about you to somebody else when you were within earshot: "She's a little fatty—she eats like a pig"; "He always falls over his own feet"; "He's such a handful—I can't stand being with him too long"; "Don't listen to her. She lies all the time." As a parent you *need* to think before you blurt something out, in order to minimize these hurt feelings that you didn't really mean to hurt at all. What do you want *your* child to remember? Think first about how you would feel if what you are about to say was said to or about you. Then decide whether or not to say it.

Unfortunately, it's also not uncommon for a parent to unintentionally dismiss his children's feelings, actions, or beliefs with statements like "What are you so scared of?"; "Be a big boy!"; "How can you do that to your sister? You're the older one!"; "Why are you always so bad?!" Negating a child, mocking him or his feelings, only encourages him to withdraw from you. Even if you don't mean to, can you see how habitually dismissing him could lead to him becoming unwilling to share his feelings with you? Your connection with him, your bond, erodes each time he feels or hears your annoyance, disdain, anger, or rejection. How can you be his guiding force if you unintentionally push him away? How can you help him to understand the world in which he has found himself if he retreats from you?

Children are very intuitive. They know, on some level, when you are being sincere with them and when you are not. Sincerity counts. If you lie to your children or mislead them, they won't trust you. They may not be aware of it on a conscious level, but there will be some sense that something is not right. This, too, will slowly erode your bond with your child. Don't promise a child anything unless you plan on fulfilling that promise; don't threaten anything unless you can and are willing to follow through with the threat. They want and need to know that you are real. Your integrity is important to both you and your child. Keeping to your word is a demonstration of that integrity.

Some children are so much more sensitive than others; they take things to heart more readily. Some don't. What is your child like? Do you know? Is she like you were as a child? Maybe she is, and maybe she's not. You'll know if you study her.

All children are naturally and quite normally self-centered. It's through their interaction with others and the world around them that they learn, over time, that they are not the center of the universe and that others' needs are just as important as their own. I've long believed that a person really becomes an adult when she has a child to raise and care for. It is only then that the self-centeredness, rooted in the child in *us*, is overcome. When you are a parent and are caring for your child, you must put aside your momentary desires and care for his needs. You are placing the baby's needs above your own, often in spite of the way you feel. You *want* to go back to sleep but you can't because the baby needs you; you *want* to take a shower, or a walk, or have a cup of coffee all by yourself, but you can't because the baby is crying or it's time to get your little one dressed and off to school. As a parent you learn to give of yourself regardless of how you feel about it. It's a marvelous growth experience for you, as a human being. If you take it on as seriously as you would your professional career or your higher education, you become a *true* adult: one who acts from what he knows in spite of what he feels.

Love

What is love? There are many different kinds: love for your parents, your siblings, your spouse, your children. Each is different from the other. But one thing is true about all of them; you only experience love, you *feel* love, when you are loving (think: action word). *It is in the act of loving that you experience the feeling of love.* You may enjoy the feeling of being loved, but you only feel love when you are doing the loving.

Many of us have experienced the unabated adoration that welled up completely unexpectedly when we saw, felt, held our babies for the first time. That wellspring of love is a gift from the Universe or God or whatever you call the Higher force with which we are permeated. That experience teaches us just how deep is our capacity to love. You build upon this pool of inner love and use it as a resource. It is what you call upon within yourself at 4 am when your baby is crying and you just can't console her, or when she's wide awake at 4 am, smiling and ready to play. It's what stems the frustration and prevents you from doing harm to her. That love that a parent has for his child is a wonderful, joyful, blessed phenomenon.

But how do you direct that deep well of love you have for your child? Some give in to every whim of the child, believing that it is out of love that you let her eat ice cream multiple times a day because she wants it, and you can't bear to see her unhappy. But is that really love?

I believe that real love for a child combines your deep affection for your child with a great desire and need to do what is best for him, both in the short term and in the long term. How to know what is best for him? Consider not just his wants but his needs to the best of your ability, and then place his needs above your own.

For example, say your four year old loves candy. You can understand it; so do you. You have it around the house all the time because you both love it so much. Your child has gotten into the habit of pestering you for candy all day long, starting early in the morning, and you just don't want to fight with her all day. But she's got a bit of a weight problem for a four year old, and maybe one of your parents has diabetes.

Look down the road a bit. Think it through. Left to eat candy as she wishes, your child may end up with an even bigger weight problem when she's a teenager (about the worst thing that can happen to a teenage girl, from her perspective). Maybe further down the road, if she continues to eat large amounts of white sugar and white flour products, she will become a diabetic—the genetic predisposition for disease can't be denied.

So what do you do? If you are placing your child's needs above your own, you can do several things:

1. You explain that candy is a special treat, not an everyday food. Explain that it is simply not good for her to eat it, and she cannot have it whenever she wants it. You might even have to argue a bit and go through this several times a day, perhaps even for several days in a row, until she's completely clear that you are not going to change your mind.
2. You throw out all the candy in your house so she doesn't see it around. Then you stop buying it.
3. *You* stop eating candy in front of her. Candy has just become a very special treat for both of you, and perhaps, in the best of worlds, you have saved her from a road that could have led to pain and suffering due to weight and health issues for years and years to come. You've sacrificed your desire not to fight with her now for her well-being in the present, and hopefully in the future as well. And in so doing, you have practiced real love.

This happens with more than just food. We let our kids do what they want because we don't want them to be mad at us or because we feel guilty that we've been away at work too long or we're just too tired to hassle with them. The overindulgences we allow could be computer time or the television programs they watch or the friends they keep or the way they treat the babysitter. Whatever it is, ask yourself first: Where will this behavior lead? Is it in my child's best interest for me to allow it to continue? What kind of person will my child become in the long run if he continues down this road? If the answer does not please you, then call upon that wellspring of inner love and fight with your kids. Love them. Truly. For their sake.

Support

I like to refer to support as the practical counterpart of a parent's love. To me, support is demonstrating that you will always be there to help your child, whenever he needs you, whatever the circumstances. Being supportive of your child builds and then strengthens his sense of self as well as his trust in you. It begins in infancy—that cry from the crib, that calling out for comfort. When you answer it your children begin to learn that you will be there for them; they learn that they can trust you, that they aren't alone, that you are there to help them, care for them, aid them no matter what they need or when they need it. It is exactly that bond of trust that you want to evolve over the years so that when your children reach their teens and experiment with alcohol for the first time with their friends, and perhaps overdo it a bit, it is *you* they call at 1 am to come and pick them up.

Mutual respect is the groundwork for that relationship. A child is a precious gift who deserves to be loved and appreciated. As a parent you need to understand that you *chose* to bring this entity into the world. You wanted a child. Again, put yourself into your child's shoes—it's not that hard, we were all children at one time. When your three year old is "helping" you wash the dishes, from his perspective he is truly helping you and he is proud of the work that he is doing. Yes, there is water going everywhere, and it will take you twice as long to clean the kitchen, but you said it was okay for him to help; he is helping. That his little hands are not quite able to do things efficiently does not diminish the effort he is making. Support his efforts, appreciate them, thank him; allow him to feel pride in his accomplishment.

When you encourage your child's efforts and help him to succeed in a new striving, he gains both a real sense of self worth and the understanding that you want him to succeed. Truly helping him to succeed does not mean doing his homework for him, and it isn't telling him that he's too young or too small to try something that he strongly desires. It's giving him the opportunity to try. It's teaching him that if at first he fails at something he wants to succeed at (which is likely to be the case—isn't it that way for us all?), he needs to practice. It's getting him to understand that he can strengthen and better himself through his own efforts, and it is providing the opportunities for him to make those efforts on his own—with your encouragement.

The other side of the coin is equally important. Try to understand your child's inherent limitations. If you are encouraging your child to go beyond what she has already accomplished, make sure that she is emotionally and developmentally ready to take that step. Don't push your child to walk if she cannot sit or crawl. Don't ask him to play his violin for the family if it will make him uncomfortable. Frustration and self-deprecation are brought into being when we are faced with doing a task that we are as yet incapable of succeeding at.

Whether you are supporting your child as he takes his first step or when you are teaching him to drive, your attitude is basically the same: I am here to help you be the best you can be, and I will always be here as long as you need me.

In supporting your child, what you are practicing is respect for your child's sovereignty as a human being. Ultimately you are helping him to be independent and self-sufficient. Isn't that the very thing that we as parents are fundamentally striving toward?

Guidance

When asked by an adult friend what prevented a child from getting involved in drugs/alcohol/bad friendships, my son replied that it was having a close relationship with his family. We spent a lot of time together, as much as we could given the fact that my husband, Steve, and I both had active professional lives, and Mark was in school and had a busy after-school schedule. We had dinners together far more often than not, and most evenings Mark spent at home with at least one parent. These were not special hours that we set aside to be together. They were the hours that we were simply together—eating dinner, watching television, cleaning the kitchen, sharing his bath-time and bedtime rituals. But Steve and I together were committed to being with Mark when we were with Mark. That is, we tried to be there for him emotionally, paying attention to him. To the best of our ability we left work at work; we discussed our personal issues when we were alone; we tried to make each of our family moments what could be called quality family time. Truth be told, for me it was a pleasure.

What constitutes "quality" family time? I think there's a general misconception that quality time involves pre-planned events, but really quality time together can be garnered from within everyday moments. Driving in the car together, even for a fifteen- or twenty-minute commute, offers a perfect opportunity to talk to one another. That's time enough to talk about lots of things: "What happened in school? How was your math test? Did you enjoy dance today? No. Why not?" It's time like that that can be used to share and learn about one another.

Consider the father who is talking on the cell phone while he is pushing his daughter on a swing or going to the grocery store with her. He's not spending time with his child. He's doing business on the phone while feeling justified in the belief that he's taking care of her. What is he missing? The utter joy of sharing in his child's delight as the swing goes higher and higher. He doesn't realize that he could be sharing in that delight just by watching it. What is she missing? A chance to talk to and get to know her daddy. How many of us didn't really know what kind of people our parents were until we were well into our adult years? What a pity.

Quality time can be found in all of the individual moments strung together over the course of the very few years that you have your child living in your home with you. It's often during those minutes that you are quietly guiding your child.

I believe that the old adage "Do as I say, not as I do" is a vastly mistaken directive. I also believe that far more important than the type of work you do is the kind of human being you are. Children learn through example. They are like little sponges, soaking up everything they see and hear. You—in your actions, your speech, your concerns, in who and what you are—are setting an example for your children to follow. When you see your child mirroring your behavior and your speech, what will you see? Guiding your child is as much about you as it is about him.

For me, it is so important to instill the seed of love for Mother Earth, Gaia, for the natural world of which we are a part. We are just a fragment, a tiny component, of that whole. Given that belief, I think that it is necessary to show our children respect for all living things: animals, plants, and our Great Mother, the ground upon which we live, Mother Earth. We are part of a vast universe that holds amazing wonders that we sometimes fail to see.

I remember when my infant granddaughter, at just a few weeks old, started seeing the world around her. She seemed to be so amazed she was unwilling to sleep. If we see these wonders, we need to show them to our children. How do you see the natural world? How do you care for the animals that share your home? The squirrels and birds that live in your yard? The local water supply? What do your children hear when you are talking about your parents, your siblings, their teachers, their friends, your friends? If your children see you acting as a caring and supportive human being, and if you teach them to think about the needs of all others creatures, you will be guiding them toward becoming that as well.

Then there are the everyday actions that guide in their own ways. I remember the first time I made a baked potato for Mark when he was tiny. I started to put butter and salt on it, just the same way as I would for myself. Then it occurred to me—if he doesn't start out eating sugars and salt, he may not develop a taste for them. So I adjusted my way of preparing food for him (and for me, by the way), eliminating the salt and the butter on that potato that night. Sure enough. He likes the taste of the food itself—not the seasonings that transform it.

We can easily define the way our children eat—with the first foods that you give to your child, you are training his palate. Think twice before allowing your child to eat highly sugared or salted foods, foods that are high in fats, or junk foods, foods that contain artificial ingredients, chemicals, or preservatives. (I do believe that if you can't pronounce an ingredient, you shouldn't eat it.) Offer him whole grains, fruits and vegetables in season, poultry, fish, beef and pork, eggs, low fat dairy products, purified water. Feed your child as you'd want him to eat for a lifetime. Over the years I've met numerous parents who are very careful about the foods that they allow their children to eat, but are not nearly as watchful of their own diet. Feed yourself as well as you feed your children—and with good fortune you will be healthy and strong as you watch your children bring up their children.

In that same vein, how much exercise do you get? How much exercise do you believe you should get? Encourage your kids to get out and exercise. Physical exertion is essential to the proper functioning of the body for both children and adults. Whether it's riding a bike or running around with the other kids in the neighborhood, going for a long walk or hike, playing ball, or swimming, dancing, skating, or doing martial arts, encourage your kids to find the joy of exercise. And join them. It's fun.

Just about everyone these days knows that you can spend way too much time sitting. Whether you're in front of a computer monitor or television screen, sitting in front of it for too long is tough on your body, your eyes, and your mind. Letting your kids spend too much time on the computer (especially without knowing what sites they are visiting or participating in) is not a great idea. The same can be said about letting them play hours of video games. Yes, those games are great for developing eye-hand coordination, but they are too often violent in nature. And somehow hours of violent, explicit television does not seem to be the best way for your child to learn about the nature of the world in which he lives. (If television and movies actually mirror our life and society, then we desperately need to change things.)

We are setting forth the course upon which our kids will walk for a long time to come, both emotionally and physically. We need to think about what we do and how we are doing it. We try to guide our children thoughtfully, carefully. We try because of the deep, unending fountain of love we have for them. All we want is for our children to be happy. But sometimes what makes *us* happy is not what makes *them* happy. We have to understand that our children will have their own personal preferences that we need to respect. Each will have her or his own life; each needs to live that life authentically, and we need to trust the choices our children make. Their lessons will be their lessons. We cannot save them from the hurts that they will inevitably encounter. But we can help them learn to be the kind of people who will be able to weather whatever storms they must encounter during the course of their lives, learning about life and about themselves from whatever comes their way.

Khalil Gibran, the Lebanese prophet, expressed this thought most beautifully. He wrote: "Your children are not your children. . . . They come through you . . . yet they belong not to you. . . . You are the bows from which your children as living arrows are sent forth."* Guide your children, care for them, love them, support them, but understand that you do not own them; nor they, you. You are forever connected, yet each is individual, like fingers on a hand. When it's time to let them go, let them go. Let them be the adults that they are. Respect them for who they have become.

And enjoy that phase, too. It's all part of the passage.

Afterword

Memo from a Child to Parents

Twenty-five or more years ago I found this in the newspaper, in an advertisement for a local health club. The ad read: "The writer of the message above is unfortunately unknown to me for credit. I found it cut out of wherever it had appeared many years ago. My children are grown up now and unfortunately I have been guilty of many of the requests in this message. I believe in this advice. More than I hope that you'll join the club, I hope you'll cut this out for when your children are growing up."

I followed the suggestion—I cut it out when my child was growing up. I pass it on to you, should you wish to do the same. In the years since I came across it, I've pondered the contents of this memo and its meaning many times.

Memo from a Child to Parents

1. Don't spoil me. I know quite well that I ought not to have all I ask for—I'm only testing you.
2. Don't be afraid to be firm with me. I prefer it. It makes me feel secure.
3. Don't let me form bad habits. I have to rely on you to detect them in the early stages.
4. Don't make me feel smaller than I am. It only makes me behave stupidly "big."
5. Don't correct me in front of people if you can help it. I'll take much more notice if you talk quietly with me in private.

6. Don't make me feel that my mistakes are sins. It upsets my sense of values.

7. Don't protect me from consequences. I need to learn the painful way sometimes.

8. Don't be too upset when I say "I hate you." Sometimes it isn't you I hate but your power to thwart me.

9. Don't take too much notice of my small ailments. Sometimes they get me the attention I need.

10. Don't nag. If you do, I shall have to protect myself by appearing deaf.

11. Don't forget that I cannot explain myself as well as I should like. That is why I am not always accurate.

12. Don't put me off when I ask questions. If you do, you will find that I stop asking and seek my information elsewhere.

13. Don't be inconsistent. That completely confuses me and makes me lose faith in you.

14. Don't tell me my fears are silly. They are terribly real and you can do much to reassure me if you try to understand.

15. Don't ever suggest that you are perfect or infallible. It gives me too great a shock when I discover that you are neither.

16. Don't ever think that it is beneath your dignity to apologize to me. An honest apology makes me feel surprisingly warm towards you.

17. Don't forget I love experimenting. I couldn't get along without it, so please put up with it.

18. Don't forget how quickly I am growing up. It must be very difficult for you to keep pace with me, but please try.

19. Don't forget that I don't thrive without lots of love and understanding, but I don't need to tell you, do I?

20. Please keep yourself fit and healthy. I need you.

Appendix

Commonly Used Acupoints

In this index, precise acupoint location is offered for those who are familiar with anatomical terminology. These are the anatomical specifics that practitioners of Oriental medicine need to know in order to be precise in their placement of acupuncture needles. Note that the standard unit of measurement in Oriental healing arts is the *tsun*. It uses the width of the thumb or length of the center phalange of the middle finger *of the person being treated* to determine accurate point location.

The acupoints listed in this appendix are those that are used most often during the course of the treatments detailed in this book.

Commonly used points of the Arm Great Yin Lung Channel (Lu)

Lu 1: On the lateral aspect of the chest, 6 tsun from the midline, in the first intercostal space

Lu 2: Below the lateral aspect of the clavicle, 6 tsun from the midline, in the deltopectoral triangle

Lu 5: At the cubital crease, lateral to the tendon of the biceps brachii muscle

Lu 6: On the radial forearm, 5 tsun below Lu 5

Lu 7: At the styloid process, 1.5 tsun above the transverse wrist crease

Lu 9: At the transverse wrist crease, in the depression on the radial side of the radial artery

Lu 10: In the center of the first metacarpal bone on the thenar eminence, where the skin of the palm meets the skin of the dorsal surface of the hand

Lu 11: On the radial side of the thumb, .1 tsun proximal to the corner of the root of the nail

Commonly used points
of the Arm Bright Yang Colon Channel (Co)

Co 1: On the radial side of the index finger, .1 tsun proximal to the corner of the root of the nail

Co 2: On the radial side of the index finger, immediately distal to the meta-carpophalangeal joint

Co 4: In the center of the second metacarpal bone, on its radial side

Co 11: In the depression formed when the elbow is flexed slightly, at the lateral end of the cubital crease, between Lu 5 and the lateral epicondyle of the humerus

Co 20: Beside the midpoint of the nasal ala in the nasolabial groove

Commonly used points
of the Leg Bright Yang Stomach Channel (St)

St 1: Between the midpoint of the infraorbital ridge and the eyeball

St 9: On a horizontal line with the thyroid cartilage (Adam's apple), at the anterior border of the sternocleidomastoid muscle

St 10: At the anterior border of the sternocleidomastoid muscle, midway between St 9 and St 11

St 11: Below St 10, superior to the clavicle, between the sternal and clavicular heads of the sternocleidomastoid muscle

St 12: At the midpoint of the supraclavicular fossa, on the mammilary line

St 25: 2 tsun lateral to the umbilicus

St 36: 3 tsun below the distal margin of the patella, 1 finger breadth lateral to the crest of the tibia

St 37: 3 tsun below St 36

St 40: 5 tsun below St 36, 1 tsun lateral to the crest of the tibia

St 43: In the depression distal to the junction of the second and third meta-tarsal bones

St 44: Distal to the second metatarsophalangeal joint, proximal to the web margin between the second and third toes

Commonly used points
of the Leg Great Yin Spleen Channel (Sp)

Sp 3: Proximal and inferior to the head of the first metatarsal bone at the medial aspect of the foot

Sp 4: Distal and inferior to the base of the first metatarsal bone at the medial aspect of the foot

Sp 6: 3 tsun proximal to the tip of the medial malleolus, on the posterior border of the tibia

Sp 10: 2 tsun proximal to the mediosuperior border of the patella, in the center of the fleshy mass of the medial quadriceps muscle, vastus medialis

Sp 11: 6 tsun proximal to Sp 10

Sp 21: 6 tsun distal to the axilla on the midaxillary line in the sixth intercostal space

Commonly used points of the Arm Lesser Yin Heart Channel (He)

He 3: At the medial end of the transverse cubital crease, located when the arm is flexed

He 6: On the ulnar side of the wrist, .5 tsun proximal to the wrist crease, radial to the tendon of flexor carpi ulnaris

He 7: On the ulnar side of the wrist crease, proximal to the pisiform bone, radial to the tendon of the flexor carpi ulnaris

He 8: On the surface of the palm in between the fourth and fifth metacarpal bones, where the tip of the pinky rests when a loose fist is made

He 9: On the radial side of the pinky, .1 tsun proximal to the corner of the root of the nail

Commonly used points of the Arm Great Yang Small Intestine Channel (SI)

SI 17: Posterior to the angle of the mandible, anterior to the sternocleido-mastoid muscle

SI 19: In the depression formed when the mouth is opened, anterior to the tragus of the ear

Commonly used points of the Leg Great Yang Bladder Channel (Bl)

Bl 1: .1 tsun superior to the inner canthus of the eye

Bl 2: At the medial end of the eyebrow in the supraorbital notch

Bl 12: 1.5 tsun lateral to the lower border of the spinous process of the second thoracic vertebra

Bl 13: 1.5 tsun lateral to the lower border of the spinous process of the third thoracic vertebra

Bl 15: 1.5 tsun lateral to the lower border of the spinous process of the fifth thoracic vertebra

Bl 17: 1.5 tsun lateral to the lower border of the spinous process of the seventh thoracic vertebra

Bl 18: 1.5 tsun lateral to the lower border of the spinous process of the ninth thoracic vertebra

Bl 20: 1.5 tsun lateral to the lower border of the spinous process of the eleventh thoracic vertebra

Bl 21: 1.5 tsun lateral to the lower border of the spinous process of the twelfth thoracic vertebra

Bl 22: 1.5 tsun lateral to the lower border of the spinous process of the first lumbar vertebra

Bl 23: 1.5 tsun lateral to the lower border of the spinous process of the second lumbar vertebra

Bl 25: 1.5 tsun lateral to the lower border of the spinous process of the fourth lumbar vertebra

Bl 26: 1.5 tsun lateral to the lower border of the spinous process of the fifth lumbar vertebra

Bl 28: Level with the second sacral foramen, in the depression between the medial border of the posterior superior iliac spine (PSIS) and the sacrum

Bl 34: In the fourth sacral foramen, 1.5 tsun lateral to midline

Bl 39: At the lateral end of the popliteal crease, medial to the tendon of biceps femoris

Bl 52: 3 tsun lateral to the lower border of the spinous process of the second lumbar vertebra

Bl 58: On the posterior border of the fibula, on the anterolateral border of gastrocnemius, 7 tsun proximal to the medial aspect of the calcaneous

Bl 63: Anterior and inferior to the tip of the lateral malleolus, in the depression inferior to the cuboid bone

Bl 64: Posterior to the tuberosity of the fifth metatarsal on the lateral aspect of the foot

Bl 65: Proximal to the head of the fifth metatarsal on the lateral aspect of the foot

Bl 66: Distal and slightly inferior to the fifth metatarsophalangeal joint

Bl 67: On the lateral aspect if the small toe, .1 tsun proximal to the corner of the root of the nail

Commonly used points of the Leg Lesser Yin Kidney Channel (Ki)

Ki 3: In the depression located midway between the tip of the medial malleolus and the Achilles tendon

Ki 6: 1 tsun below the medial malleolus

Ki 7: 2 tsun proximal to Ki 3, at the anterior border of the Achilles tendon

Ki 16: .5 tsun lateral to the umbilicus

Ki 22: In the fifth intercostal space 2 tsun lateral to the midline

Ki 23: In the fourth intercostal space 2 tsun lateral to the midline

Ki 24: In the third intercostal space 2 tsun lateral to the midline

Ki 25: In the second intercostal space, 2 tsun lateral to the midline

Ki 26: In the first intercostal space 2 tsun lateral to the midline

Commonly used points
of the Arm Absolute Yin Pericardium Channel (PC)

PC 3: In the center of the transverse cubital crease on the ulnar side of the tendon of the biceps brachii muscle

PC 5: 3 tsun proximal to the transverse wrist crease between the tendons of palmaris longus and flexor carpi radialis

PC 6: 2 tsun proximal to the transverse wrist crease between the tendons of palmaris longus and flexor carpi radialis

PC 7: At the transverse wrist crease between the tendons of palmaris longus and flexor carpi ulnaris

PC 8: In the center of the palm between the second and third metacarpal bones proximal to the third metacarpophalangeal joint

PC 9: On the radial side of the middle finger, .1 tsun proximal to the corner of the root of the nail

Commonly used points
of the Arm Lesser Yang Triple Warmer Channel (TW)

TW 3: On the dorsum of the hand, proximal to the fourth metacarpophalangeal joint

TW 5: 2 tsun above the transverse crease of the dorsal wrist between the radius and the ulna

TW 6: 3 tsun above the transverse crease of the dorsal wrist between the radius and the ulna

TW 17: In the space between the angle of the mandible and the mastoid process behind the ear lobe

TW 21: In the depression formed when the mouth is opened anterior and superior to the tragus of the ear directly above SI 19

Commonly used points
of the Leg Lesser Yang Gall Bladder Channel (GB)

GB 2: In the depression formed when the mouth is opened, inferior and anterior to the tragus of the ear directly below SI 19

GB 11: Posterior to the ear, superior to the mastoid process, on a horizontal line with the tragus of the ear

GB 14: On the forehead, 1 tsun above the midpoint of the eyebrow

GB 20: At the base of the occiput, between the attachment of the sterno-cleidomastoid muscle and upper trapezius

GB 21: At the high point of the muscle mass at the midpoint of the upper shoulder, midway between the spinous process of the sixth cervical vertebra and the acromion

Commonly used points of the
Leg Absolute Yin Liver Channel (Liv)

Liv 2: Distal to the metacarpophalangeal joint of the great toe, proximal to the web margin

Liv 3: Distal to the base of the first metatarsal bone

Liv 5: 5 tsun above the tip of the medial malleolus on the posterior border of the tibia

Liv 8: At the medial end of the popliteal fold, posterior to the medial condyle of the tibia at the anterior border of the tendons of semitendinosus and semimembranosus

Liv 9: 4 tsun proximal to the medial epicondyle of the femur, between vastus medialis and sartorius

Commonly used points
of the Conception Vessel (CV)

CV 3: On the anterior midline, 1 tsun above the pubic symphysis, 4 tsun below the umbilicus

CV 4: On the anterior midline, 3 tsun below the umbilicus

CV 6: On the anterior midline, 1.5 tsun below the umbilicus

CV 10: On the anterior midline, 2 tsun above the umbilicus

CV 11: On the anterior midline, 3 tsun above the umbilicus

CV 12: On the anterior midline, 4 tsun above the umbilicus

CV 13: On the anterior midline, 5 tsun above the umbilicus

CV 14: On the anterior midline, 6 tsun above the umbilicus

CV 15: On the anterior midline, 7 tsun above the umbilicus; most often located just distal to the xyphoid process

CV 17: On the anterior midline, midway between the nipples at the level of the fourth intercostal space

Commonly used Extra Points

Yintang: On the anterior midline of the face, midway between the eyebrows

Taiyang: In the depression on the temple, 1 tsun posterior to the midpoint between the lateral end of the eyebrow and the outer canthus

Bitong: In the depression below the nasal bone superior to the nasal ala

Resources

We live in an age where massive amounts of information on every subject imaginable are available twenty-four hours a day via the Internet. In my mind this is a double-edged sword. On the one hand, the information is there to be consumed; on the other, not everything you find on the Internet is useful or valuable. Sometimes taken out of context, bits of information can be misunderstood.

Also, textbook descriptions of illness rarely occur. Most illnesses are variations on a theme, variations that are dependent on individual differences: age, family history, health background, diet, and exercise patterns, to name but a few. Gather your information from the Internet if you choose to do so, but don't let that replace working with a health professional or medical doctor who you know and trust and who will see and appreciate your child for the individual he or she is.

The websites that do the best job regarding children's health conditions are those that provide easy-to-understand, useful, well-balanced information and advice. The following is a sampling of those types of websites.

The last two websites provide information about protecting our environment and keeping our foods safe and healthy. When it comes right down to it, when we work in concert with Mother Earth we ultimately invest in our children's health and well-being.

Virtual Pediatric Hospital
http://www.virtualpediatrichospital.org/
    I use this site to...

Mayo Clinic

http://www.mayoclinic.com/health/childrens-health/CC99999

The Children's Hospital of Philadelphia

http://www.chop.edu/consumer/your_child/wellness_index.jsp

Ask Doctor Sears

http://askdrsears.com/html/10/index.asp

Keep Kids Healthy.com

http://www.keepkidshealthy.com/welcome/welcome.html

KidsHealth

http://kidshealth.org/parent/

Parent's Common Sense Encyclopedia

http://www.drhull.com/EncyMaster/index.html

Cincinnati Children's

http://www.cincinnatichildrens.org/health/info/

Natural Resources Defense Council

http://nrdc.org/

Center for Science in the Public Interest

http://www.cspinet.org/

Bibliography

Brace, Edward R., and John P. Pacanowski, MD. *Childhood Symptoms*. New York: Stonesong Press, 1985.

Chen, Jing. *Anatomical Atlas of Chinese Acupuncture Points*. Jinan, China: Shandong Science and Technology Press, 1988.

Eisenberg, Arlene, Heidi Murkoff, and Sandee Hathaway. *What to Expect the First Year*. New York: Workman Publishing, 1996.

Ellis, Andrew, Nigel Wiseman, and Ken Boss. *Fundamentals of Chinese Acupuncture*. Taos, N.Mex.: Paradigm Publications, 1991.

Finando, Donna. *Trigger Point Self Care Manual*. Rochester, Vt.: Healing Arts Press, 2006

Finando, Donna, and Steven Finando. *Trigger Point Therapy for Myofascial Pain*. Rochester, Vt.: Healing Arts Press, 2005.

Gibran, Khalil. *The Prophet*. New York: Alfred A. Knopf, 1923.

Hseuh, Chen Chiu. *Acupunture, A Comprehensive Text*. Translated and edited by John O'Connor and Dan Bensky, Shanghai College of Traditional Medicine. Seattle: Eastland Press, 1981.

Karp, M.D., Harvey. *The Happiest Baby on the Block*. New York: Bantam Dell, 2002.

Leach, Penelope. *Your Baby and Child*, 3rd ed. New York: Alfred A. Knopf, 2000.

Louv, Richard. *Last Child in the Woods*. Chapel Hill, N.C.: Algonquin Books, 2006.

Maciocia, Giovanni. *The Foundations of Chinese Medicine*. Edinburgh: Churchill Livingstone, 1989.

———. *The Practice of Chinese Medicine*. Edinburgh: Churchill Livingstone, 1994.

O'Connor, John, and Dan Bensky. *Acupuncture, A Comprehensive Text*. Seattle: Eastland Press, 1985.

Schiff, Donald, M.D., and Steven P. Shevlov, M.D., eds. *American Academy of Pediatrics Guide to Your Child's Symptoms*. New York: Villard Books (Random House), 1997.

Silver, Henry K., M.D, et. al. *Handbook of Pediatrics*. Norwalk, Conn.: Appleton and Lange, 1987.

Simons, David, Janet Travell, and Lois Simons. *Travell and Simons' Myofascial Pain and Dysfunction, The Trigger Point Manual*, volume I, 2nd ed. Baltimore: Williams and Wilkins, 1999.

Sohn, Tina, and Donna Finando. *Amma: The Ancient Art of Oriental Healing.* Rochester, Vt.: Healing Arts Press, 1988.

Spock, Benjamin, M.D., *Dr. Spock's The First Two Years.* New York: Simon and Schuster, 2001.

Spock, Benjamin, M.D., and Michael Rothenberg, M.D. *Dr. Spock's Baby and Child Care.* New York: Simon and Schuster, 1985.

Tortora, Gerard, and Nicholas Anagnostakos. *Principles of Anatomy and Physiology.* New York: Harper and Row, 1981.

Travell, Janet, and David Simons. *Myofascial Pain and Dysfunction: The Trigger Point Manual,* volume II. Baltimore: Williams and Wilkins, 1992.

Upledger, John, and Jon Vredevoogd. *Craniosacral Therapy.* Seattle: Eastland, 1983.

Zand, Janet, L.Ac., O.M.D. *Smart Medicine for a Healthier Child.* New York: Avery Publishing, 1994.

Essentials of Chinese Acupuncture. Beijing: Foreign Languages Press, 1980.

An Outline of Chinese Acupuncture. Peking: Foreign Languages Press, 1975.

Index